An Intersectional Guide for Male Survivors of Sexual Abuse and Their Allies

Few experiences carry more shame, stigma, and misunderstanding than the life-altering trauma of sexual abuse. Men who experience sexual abuse and rape, often find themselves marginalised and isolated, yet there are few resources available for them or those who support them.

This book examines the impact of sexual abuse on different men through an intersectional lens, exploring how their unique identities, circumstances, and society's views affect their recovery or compound their trauma. Each chapter addresses a topic chosen by hundreds of male survivors who have attended the author's recovery groups. It includes survivor testimonies, signposts to resources, and reflective activities to help manage the aftermath of sexual trauma. With statutory services, such as the criminal justice system, often failing male survivors, the book draws on Transformative Justice principles to suggest alternative ways for men to break cycles of trauma and move forward with their lives.

Aimed at male survivors and those who support them – counsellors, psychotherapists, social workers, family members, and loved ones – this book offers guidance and hope for navigating a path to healing.

Jeremy Sachs is a therapist from London, now based in Glasgow. Since the 2010s, he has run services that support individuals living with trauma or marginalisation, helping them to connect and find community. In 2016, he focused on developing therapy services for men, boys, and trans people who have survived sexual abuse and rape. He runs recovery groups and a private practice both online and in-person, and is a trustee at Wellbeing Scotland.

@JeremySachs_
@jeremysachs.bsky.social
www.jeremysachs.com

'Packed full of insights, practical guidance and signposting, this is an engaging, accessible, and deeply compassionate text for male survivors of sexual abuse and their allies—including the professionals working with them. An essential guide for those wanting to navigate this complex, sensitive, but profoundly important field.'
Mick Cooper, *author of* Psychology at the Heart of Social Change
(Policy Press, 2023)

'Jeremy Sachs' thoughtful, caring and sensitive exploration of the complexities and nuances of the under-recognised impact of male sexual trauma and abuse will benefit men, their allies, and clinicians in navigating words and experiences hidden by years of emotional turmoil. This essential resource will assist in demystifying survivors' experiences.'
Andrew Davidson, *Joint Programme Head of the Diploma in Psychosexual Therapy at Tavistock Relationships*

'This book shares a rare combination of personal insight and professional experience that will benefit everyone affected by sexual violence against men and boys. This is the sort of book that you do not read just once. Instead, you can keep it with you, returning to it as different challenges emerge and subside, knowing that each time you open it you will find something to help you through.'
Tanaka Mhishi, *Author of* Sons and Others: On Loving Male Survivors

Given that patriarchal adaptations mean men are often taught to hide, or suppress, the shame of sexual abuse, to have so gentle, yet so pointed and strong, a masculine voice speak on so sensitive a subject says a lot about the power of the prose presented in this volume. This is an emotional, sensitive tome, written from the thoughtful and somatically considered. This book lays out that road, presents pathways for practitioners to work with what is a challenging, little understood, yet hugely important experience for a good number of men. This is therefore a worthwhile, easy to access, deep dive into the experiences of male survivors of sexual abuse, which offers routes forward for practitioners working with these issues in their practices.'
Dr Dwight Turner, *(He/Him), PhD, Dipl Supvn, Psychotherapist, Supervisor, and Workshop, Facilitator, UKCP Accredited*

'As a survivor of sexual violence who has also worked extensively with other survivors, I was delighted to see this comprehensive yet accessible guide for male survivors and their allies. Jeremy brings a wealth of knowledge and experience and communicates this, through the book, in a way that will resonate with male survivors, whatever their background or experience of sexual violence. It speaks directly to the challenges we all face as we heal and guides the reader through a range of exercises to support the process. Reading this guide took me to a warm place of comfort and reflection and I know it will be life-changing for many male survivors.'

Alex Feis-Bryce, *CEO Diversity Role Models*

'*An Intersectional Guide for Male Survivors of Sexual Abuse and Their Allies* is profoundly moving: emotionally, it draws you into the embodied narratives of male sexual abuse survivors, compelling you to immerse in their lived realities often shrouded in silence. Conceptually, it challenges the very core of persistent myths about what it means to live as, and be, a man. Therapeutically, it provokes a necessary and urgent reckoning amongst mental health professionals, urging us to question how rigid social construc-tions of masculinity implicitly guide therapeutic interactions with male ser-vice users, where silent struggles may be mistaken as stoic endurance.

Dr Nini Kerr, *Senior Lecturer in Counselling, Psychotherapy and Applied Social Sciences, School of Health in Social Science, The University of Edinburgh*

'In this book, Jeremy Sachs engages the reader with essential information, practical guidance and real-life examples, supported by reflective activities and resources. The emphasis on the impact of intersectionality provides a contemporary and much-needed lens through which to understand the unique difficulties of male survivors. But it is the way that Jeremy writes, making the reader feel understood, supported, and respected, that gives a sense that he is there with you throughout.'

Professor Kate Smith, *University of Aberdeen*

'Jeremy has written a profoundly, deeply insightful book that is woven with a wisdom that inspires one's journey to transform trauma into triumph. It is a road map that enables one's own critical reflections to invite personal trans-formation which in turn has the capacity to create societal transformation.'

Arthur Lockhart, *Order of Ontario, Founder of The Gatehouse, Toronto & Co-founder of the Survivors Council Canada*

An Intersectional Guide for Male Survivors of Sexual Abuse and Their Allies

Masculinity Reconnected

Jeremy Sachs

Illustrations by Jeremy Sachs

Routledge
Taylor & Francis Group

LONDON AND NEW YORK

Designed cover image: Cover illustration by George Douglas

First published 2026
by Routledge
4 Park Square, Milton Park, Abingdon, Oxon OX14 4RN

and by Routledge
605 Third Avenue, New York, NY 10158

Routledge is an imprint of the Taylor & Francis Group, an informa business

© 2026 Jeremy Sachs

British Library Cataloguing-in-Publication Data
A catalogue record for this book is available from the British Library

Library of Congress Cataloging-in-Publication Data
Names: Sachs, Jeremy author
Title: An intersectional guide for male survivors of sexual abuse and their allies : masculinity reconnected / Jeremy Sachs ; illustrations by Jeremy Sachs.
Description: Abingdon, Oxon ; New York : Routledge, 2025. |
Includes bibliographical references and index. |
Identifiers: LCCN 2024060330 (print) | LCCN 2024060331 (ebook) |
ISBN 9781032729831 hardback | ISBN 9781032721903 paperback |
ISBN 9781003423331 ebook
Subjects: LCSH: Male sexual abuse victims—Psychology |
Male sexual abuse victims—Counseling of—Great Britain
Classification: LCC RC560.S44 S23 2025 (print) | LCC RC560.S44 (ebook) |
DDC 362.8830811—dc23/eng/20250519
LC record available at https://lccn.loc.gov/2024060330
LC ebook record available at https://lccn.loc.gov/2024060331

ISBN: 978-1-032-72983-1 (hbk)
ISBN: 978-1-032-72190-3 (pbk)
ISBN: 978-1-003-42333-1 (ebk)

DOI: 10.4324/9781003423331

Typeset in Times New Roman
by Newgen Publishing UK

Contents

Thanks and acknowledgements

I want to acknowledge two types of privilege that have enabled the existence of this book. First, I have the privilege of having resources enough to write this book in the first place! For most of my life, I couldn't have imagined this. The book exists thanks to the privileges I am able to access at this moment in my life, such as time, emotional support, and financial security.

Second, I have the privilege of knowing the people listed below, whose support has directly or indirectly led to this publication.

Thanks to my critical friends

These are professionals, people with lived experience, or people who live and work within diverse communities who have offered feedback on various chapters of this book. You have helped guide the intersectional elements and pointed out gaps in my knowledge. I'm so grateful for your guidance. In no particular order: Olumide Ajulo, Silva Neves, Dr Dena Arya, Sonny Hallett, Chris Lavin, and Steve Fearns.

Thanks to these professionals

Thank you to Kieran McCrystal for your clinical supervision and Phil Anderson for my many years of therapy. Thanks to Grace McDonnell at Routledge and Rachel Wright for the insight and edits. Thanks to all at the Association for Young People's Health, particularly Ann Hagell and Emma Rigby, for the space to grow professionally. Thanks to Arthur Lockhart and the team at The Gatehouse, Toronto, Canada, for your belief in this project.

Thanks to my friends and chosen family

In no particular order, thanks to Eve Wallman, Dr Jen O'Sullivan, Aaron Minnigin, Ilana Winterstein, Helena Monteiro, and Ruby Cedar.

Special thanks to Katherine Cox. Working alongside and learning from you has impacted my practice, this book, and myself in countless ways. And, special thanks to Cordelia Wyche, a remarkable therapist who tirelessly re-read these chapters always offering insight, challenge, and support.

Thanks to all the survivors who have contributed to this book, both those whose testimonies are featured and those who were not able to share their stories this time.

Additional thanks to my clients of all genders, both in individual and group therapy. You have been seminal in my growth and in the development of this book. The knowledge in these pages was not sourced from textbooks but rather was found in the spaces between us and the connections we made.

Lastly, I want to acknowledge all male survivors of sexual abuse. You are not alone.

Chapter 1

Introduction

I'm glad you're here

Chapter Contents

1.1 Hello: Me, you, and how to use this book

Hello

I imagine starting to write any book is hard. However, starting to write a book about the often marginalised and stigmatised topic of sexual abuse experienced by men perhaps comes with some unique challenges. The book must be formal enough to communicate useful information, psychological insights, and psychoeducation, but feel safe enough to readers to be accessible and not overwhelming. In the sexual abuse recovery groups I run, I start the first session by introducing myself and congratulating the brave group members for attending. It seems fitting then, as the knowledge in this book is the collective wisdom of those groups, that I start this book in the same way, by introducing myself and telling you how amazing I think you are for picking it up.

Me

I'm Jeremy Sachs. I grew up in South London. I now live in Glasgow. I have German-Jewish and Irish-Catholic heritage. My early life was chaotic, followed by a period of homelessness in my twenties. I worked on building sites and in hard landscaping, then in theatre and special educational needs (SEN) schools as a teaching assistant. Somewhere in the 2010s, I started creating spaces where people who had survived trauma could meet and feel a little more connected than they were previously. The first of these groups was with homeless young people in central London. I found that as I supported the young people, their energy also nourished me. Shame I felt about my past started to recede just a little as the groups became more coherent, supportive,

DOI: 10.4324/9781003423331-1

and caring. After that, I ran projects for foreign national detainees and their families, adopted young people, and refugees. In 2015, I ran the UK's only HIV-aware youth group for 10- to 12-year-olds, as well as HIV-aware groups for 13- to 19-year-olds. At the end of 2016, the male rape and sexual abuse charity SurvivorsUK asked me to create and facilitate a new group work service with my friend and colleague Katherine Cox. SurvivorsUK had run a group years before, but I was told it hadn't been successful. The men found the process of groups too difficult, and the therapists struggled to keep the sessions psychologically safe. My aim was to create a therapeutic group that met for 12 sessions over three months. It would holistically support men, allow them to share experiences, provide psychological interventions, and reduce isolation. After two years of successfully delivering this model, I expanded its methodology to work with teenage boys who had survived sexual abuse and a group to support trans and nonbinary people who had accessed the charity.

On the first day of each new group, we agree which topics to unpack over the next 11 sessions. At the end of each weekly session, we pick one topic out of the 11 to start with the next week. This gives group members a week to think about the topic coming up and emotionally prepare for it.

Each chapter in this book reflects one of the common topics picked by the hundreds of survivors who have attended my groups. The chapter order in this book is approximately the same order in which groups usually choose to look at the topics discussed. There are obviously exceptions. However, it amazes me how hundreds of different men all decided, more or less, to discuss these topics and in this order. Despite this, it is important to remember that healing from sexual abuse is not linear. The recovery journey does not go in a straight line. It is my wish that you, as the reader, move through this book as the group members did, coming to terms with your own experience, feeling less isolated and better armed with more information on trauma and abuse to help make sense of the pain. To do this you may want to start with the chapters that feel important to you. Or you may want to start with chapters that are less emotionally charged. The book has been written assuming many will read it in order, cover to cover, but if that doesn't work for you, that's okay! Feel free to pick and choose what you read and when you read it.

Throughout the book there will be reflective activities, blank sheets for notes, exercises, and importantly, testimonies from male survivors themselves, sharing how the different themes in this book have affected their recovery. It has been a privilege to feature these men's testimonies, and I'll never have words enough to thank them for trusting me with their experiences. What I can say is that this book would not exist without them. It is essential to me that their voices be at the heart of this book so that they can be read by those who will believe them and we can learn from their bravery.

Limitations of this book

I want to acknowledge from the start that this book will have limitations. I want to acknowledge this for a few reasons. When we survive a trauma like rape or sexual abuse, it can feel like we are the only ones in the world feeling the way we do. We can have violent thoughts that scare us, do things we are ashamed of, and feel isolated from the rest of society. If our identity is also marginalised, we can feel this isolation even more strongly. I want this book to speak to as many people as want to read it, but realistically these pages will not be able to reflect all identities and experiences. This book is the start of a conversation, and I hope to see many more intersectionally focused psychology books in the future. If you feel your experience is not represented here, this does not mean you are alone or 'crazy'. It simply means this book has gaps in knowledge or limitations. One thing I *do* want to acknowledge is that psychology has failed many identities within our society. Reasons for this are multifaceted, and I will get into them later. One predominant failure, however, is that in Western therapy and self-help, a *return to safety* is often viewed as an end goal of psychological interventions. *Safety* is a place that many psychological interventions hope to return clients to after trauma. The truth is that, for many people, safety has never been a part of their lives, either before or after sexual abuse. It is not a place to return to because it never existed. For many, safety cannot exist in a society where there is structural oppression and violence towards the vulnerable and minoritised. Western medicine has been built on colonialism and the exploitation of enslaved Black bodies used for experimentation. Look no further than J. Marion Sims, often called the 'father of anaesthesia', who performed experiments on Black female slaves without anaesthesia. The field of psychology was created in this climate and its legacy lives on today in medical racism and the pathologisation of identities.

Many self-help books from well-known psychologists or coaches focus on changing your perceptions in order to find peace, happiness, or security. The ability to change perceptions is useful; it is one way in which we grow. However, this approach can miss the reality of many survivors. It puts the responsibility of feeling safe on the survivor, rather than acknowledging that for many, the world continues to be dangerous, even when the abuse is over. Additionally, even among survivors who don't face systemic oppression, many men remain in some form of relationship with a family member or other person who abused them or allowed that abuse to happen. Their world cannot be safe under these conditions.

My commitment in this book is to recognise that being a male survivor will mean different things to different people and that men from all backgrounds carry unique wounds and vulnerabilities due to how the world observes them and how they view themselves in the world. This book is not about prioritising one identity over another; it is about respecting people's uniqueness, whether that is in their experience or identity. I believe there is space for us all to heal and reconnect after trauma. In fact, I have sat in few more tolerant, generous, diverse, and curious spaces in my life than I do when I sit in a room of male sexual abuse survivors, because, as the quotation often attributed to psychologist William James says, 'We are like islands in the sea, separate on the surface but connected in the deep'.[1]

You

Sexual trauma can be catastrophic – so much so that we can take all those painful memories that seem unbearable, put them a box, and lock them away somewhere deep in our minds. And for a time, this can seem to work. We make new relationships, we work, we busy ourselves with life.

Eventually though, the psychological symptoms of sexual abuse can start to leak out of the box. These symptoms can seem like they have nothing to do with sexual trauma: pain in the body, feeling angry more often than others, difficulties with sex or sexual dysfunctions. We can pivot from complete numbness to feeling overwhelmed. Some symptoms can be behavioural, such as addictions to substances or complicated relationships with work or food. Some people stop taking care of their physical health while others can become overly dependent on wellness and healthy living.

Some of the psychological symptoms of sexual abuse, however, are clearly to do with the abuse: flashbacks, bad dreams, feeling unsafe all the time, or being triggered by smells, songs, places – even colours and textures are enough to activate someone's fight or flight response.

If you are reading this book, it is likely that the box you pushed your trauma into has started opening (or in some cases, the lid has been blown right off). Or perhaps you've chosen to return to that box in order to lift the lid and look in. Either way, part of you wants to understand your past traumas better, wants to take some control over your mental health, and perhaps, holds some hope for future you. I am full of admiration for your bravery in picking up this book. I hope some of it helps, but even if it doesn't, you have taken a step towards wanting to heal and I think that is incredible.

You may also be someone who supports a survivor of sexual abuse – an ally. This comes with its own emotional journey. You will know that sexual abuse can affect everything and everybody in a survivor's life, from the ability to attend appointments on time to the most intimate sex life. Many people, both professionals and loved ones, can feel lost, not knowing where or how to start supporting a survivor. While I have chosen to write this book primarily speaking to survivors, it's my hope this book will give you insight into what might be happening for the survivors in your life and how that may impact the support you provide them. I also hope this book will help you reflect on your own journey as an ally, what that uniquely means to you and how you manage your own wellbeing when sitting with this difficult subject.

When I think of the word 'survivor' or *survival*, I think of it as a process. In my mind I picture someone swimming to shore after a shipwreck, someone climbing a cliff face, making their way to safety. The process of surviving is the process of transitioning from one state to another: from peril to safety. To me 'surviving' doesn't have to be permanent. People can move from being victim to survivor to thriver and back again. While reading this book, you may find yourself feeling complicated emotions, moving between victim, survivor, and thriver. Sometimes it can be hard to identify these feelings, and that can leave a person exhausted, angry, frustrated, or numb. Please know this is to be expected. So many survivors have learned how to exist in crisis mode every day, sometimes for months, years, or decades. Part of the process of recovery from sexual abuse is learning that while being in crisis mode may have saved your life, it might not be necessary all the time anymore. It is my hope that this book can demonstrate some ways of being in the world that are alternatives to the state of emotional crisis in which many survivors constantly live their lives. (If you do struggle to identify strong feelings, take a look at the emotions wheel on page 256 and see if that helps put words to your feelings).

How to use this book

As a child I remember bafflement from my teachers. I couldn't spell, do joined-up handwriting, or add. My coordination, or lack of it, meant I couldn't skip rope or participate well in sport. Lots of people 'had a go' at diagnosing me with various presentations: autism, obsessive compulsive disorder (OCD), etc. By the time I was 18, the times had (somewhat) caught up, and I got the diagnoses of dyslexia, dyspraxia, and dyscalculia. Even later, in my early thirties, I realised I was a shame-prone child who would do anything to avoid talking to teachers or interacting with authority figures in case they made me feel small or stupid or threatened. All this is to say that my relationship with academia was (and continues to be) difficult. I had to find lots of alternative, creative ways to engage with reading, work, and studies. I want to invite you to be creative and compassionate to yourself as you work through these pages. Use the blank pages for note-taking, doodling, and processing. Share chapters with friends or allies. Read it from cover to cover or cherry-pick bits according to your energy and interest. It is your recovery, your journey, and your book!

In these pages, you'll find

- **Testimonies from survivors**. This element has been crucial in creating this book. Hearing directly from survivors not only provides context to the topics but also, I hope, reassures you that you are not alone.

  Some men have written their testimonies independently, while others have asked to create theirs collaboratively with me. For these, I transcribed a meeting between us and turned it into a testimony, which the survivor then read and either made changes or signed off.

  These testimonies reflect a diverse range of men's identities and experiences. To honour this diversity, I have asked each contributor how they wish to be identified. Some men have chosen to remain anonymous, while others have shared details such as their race, sexuality, class, or other aspects of their identity they felt were significant when considering intersectionality and men's experience of sexual abuse.

- **Reflective activities.** Throughout the book, I suggest activities designed to help you break down the topics covered or consider how these topics affect you personally. They range from lists of issues you might consider to simple questions to help you reflect on your experience and what it means to you.
- **Exercises.** At the end of most chapters will be exercises. These are designed to help you either manage difficult emotions or think about your recovery in different ways. Some may work for you while others won't. These are opportunities to try out different things. At the end of this book, you'll find an appendix that lists each exercise and page number so you can find them quickly if you need.
- **Resources and signposting.** At the end of most chapters, you will find resources such as books, films, and websites to further explore the issues discussed. Additionally, there will be signposting to charities and support services you may find helpful. An appendix at the end of the book includes all resources and signposting in one place. (A quick disclaimer: I have tried to ensure all external resources and signposts listed are inclusive and affirming, but I can't guarantee this).
- **Blank sheets.** These are spaces for you to use as you please. Write notes to yourself, questions for a friend or therapist, doodle or draw; it is up to you how you use these.

The golden rule is to use what is helpful and leave what is not. Who knows; what you need may change over time, so don't be afraid to return to reflective activities or exercises.

1.2   Men's health and why intersectionality is important for male survivors

It's rare that men ask for help. This, it seems, is not unique to sexual abuse, but across health more generally. Men's health and health behaviour (how they take care of themselves) tend to be poor. Data from the National Health Service (NHS), World Health Organisation (WHO), and the Office for National Statistics tell us that

- Men across all socio-economic groups demonstrate unhealthier smoking practices, unhealthier dietary patterns, higher alcohol consumption levels, and higher rates of injuries.[2]
- In the UK one man in five (19 per cent) dies before they are eligible to collect their pension.[3]
- Men are less likely than women to visit their doctor or a pharmacy. Women aged 20 to 40 see a general practitioner (GP) twice as often as men in the same age group. Additionally, men are less likely than women to acknowledge illness or seek help when sick.[4]
- Men in the UK are more likely to experience poor health outcomes for a variety of conditions such as some cancers, heart disease and type 2 diabetes.[5]

- Only 36 per cent of NHS referrals for psychological therapies are for men. Despite this, in England and Wales, males accounted for around three-quarters of suicides registered in 2022 (4,179 deaths; 74.1 per cent).[6]
- In 2022, the rate of suicide mortality in males was 2.9 times higher than the rate for females. Suicide mortality in the most deprived areas of Scotland was 2.6 times higher than that in the least deprived areas in Scotland.[7]

We know men don't engage with healthcare effectively, but what is less clear is why. Many anecdotal articles written by GPs and therapists agree that damaging societal ideas about masculinity are a big culprit. Seeking help is viewed as a weakness, and admitting to illness feels vulnerable. Many men don't want to 'bother' a doctor, and they may play down or withhold symptoms during examinations. Underneath this behaviour seems to lie a fear that a bad diagnosis would be too emotionally difficult – either an illness would be unmanly or too scary to deal with. These beliefs perpetuate poor health outcomes for men and occur in part due to damaging ideas of masculinity (see Chapter 4, page 62). Based on my experience working with men, I believe that factors beyond these damaging ideas contribute to men's poor health outcomes. Specifically, the unique barriers they face in accessing support and healthcare. To explore these issues, it can help us to look at the concept of intersectionality.

Intersectionality and why it's important for male survivors

In the late 1980s, the word *intersectionality* was coined by civil rights activist and legal scholar Kimberlé Crenshaw. She argued that traditional feminist ideas and antiracist policies exclude Black women. This is because being Black and being a woman are not separate identities, although feminist and antiracist movements at the time did not consider these two parts of Black women's identities as affecting each other or impacting the experience of discrimination. Crenshaw argued that Black women experience uniquely overlapping discrimination, making the intersectional experience greater than the sum of racism and sexism.[8] Crenshaw said, during a 2016 TED Talk called 'The urgency of intersectionality', that several social justice issues we face, such as racism and misogyny, often overlap each other, meaning social injustice becomes layered and more complex than any one type of discrimination by itself.[9] The term *intersectionality* caught on and is now used to describe how interconnected social categorisations and identities – such as class, race, gender, religion, and disability – can overlap and be used within our society as cumulative forms of discrimination and oppression.

Therapy historically focuses on the experience of the individual. The therapist tries to understand the world from their client's point of view and to empathetically help them navigate personal challenges. However, I believe intersectionality allows us to be interested in broader influences that affect mental health, such as discrimination, stigma, and oppression. These influences are experienced individually by our clients but also collectively within different communities we may work with. How survivors of sexual abuse are affected by the trauma doesn't necessarily depend solely on the severity of the abuse. The circumstances around the abuse and the support or oppression survivors face before, during, and after abuse have an impact on their ability to heal from their experience or exacerbate the symptoms of sexual trauma (see Chapter 2, page 22). Considering intersectionality can be helpful for therapists and survivors alike in understanding the unique challenges individuals and communities face.

It's common for male sexual abuse survivors to either have impostor syndrome and feel everyone else's sexual trauma is so much worse or, conversely, feel that their trauma is the most severe and that no one will be able to understand their pain. Both mindsets can prevent survivors from healing or connecting with others in their lives. I often say that there is no sense in creating a hierarchy of suffering. Everyone's experience is valid, and everyone is worthy of support, connection, and kinship. However, that does not mean everyone is the same, and this is where we can use intersectionality. A Black transgender man in their twenties will have faced different challenges than a straight white man in his forties. They are both deserving of support, but one may struggle more to find support, and the support they need may differ.

Another part of intersectionality is understanding that men are likely to have survived a variety of different painful life experiences. As I note multiple times in this book, *sexual abuse rarely happens in a vacuum*. Often there are other experiences present that can cause harm. These can include other types of abuse, such as physical violence or institutional abuse, police violence, or dismissal by medical staff. Additionally, male survivors may face challenging circumstances that can impact trauma recovery, such as poverty.

1.3   Types of abuse

Below is a list of different types of abuse, followed by a list of different types of sexual abuse. The list format may imply such types of abuse occur separately from each other. However, this is not necessarily the case for survivors. Domestic abuse is often accompanied by sexual abuse, financial abuse with coercive control, and neglect with emotional abuse. Those in abusive relationships often experience various abuses that merge into one awful, traumatic experience.

This list is not exhaustive; you may have experienced or know of a type of abuse not mentioned here. However, my hope is that the list of different forms of abuse will not only help you feel better able to identify the sexual abuse you have survived, but it will also give you more information about the types of abuse that people can be vulnerable to. Do take care of yourself as you read this. Emotions can creep up on us even when reading about abuses we have not experienced. Use the blank space at the end of this chapter for notes and try out the grounding exercises, (see page 254), if you start to feel overwhelmed.

Some common types of abuse

Physical

Physical abuse is the use or threat of force by one person to control another. It is often assumed that the abuser using force is bigger or stronger than the victim. This is not always the case: a smaller, less physically strong person can physically abuse a bigger or stronger person.

Emotional

Emotional abuse can involve putting down, insulting, or shaming another person or making them feel small, scared, or vulnerable. It is often used as a weapon to undermine the victim, as well as keeping them in their relationship with the abuser. This can also be part of bullying and is often overlooked, particularly in childhood and adolescence, when bullying is considered part of growing up rather than abuse.

Neglect

Neglect is well known for being overlooked or hard to prove in statutory bodies or courts. It often consists of the failure of someone in a caring role to meet the care needs of someone else. This may be a child, an older person, or someone who lacks control over their lives. Not only can neglect be hard to prove, but it can also be one of the most harmful experiences for children. It is often hard for adults who experienced neglect as a child to recover from it or even recognise it as an issue.

Parental alienation

Parental alienation is a strategy whereby one parent deliberately intentionally tries to negatively influence or damage a child's relationship with the other parent. This can also be considered emotional child abuse and part of domestic abuse towards a partner or spouse.

Financial

Financial abuse involves controlling or stealing another person's money or resources. This can be done explicitly or implicitly with the intent to control a person or limit their freedom. It can also be a type of coercive control.

Coercive control

Coercive control is the use of mental and emotional control to limit someone's freedom of choice or thought or to get them to act or perform in ways they do not want to. The term 'gaslighting' is used to describe the ways in which someone can manipulate reality so that another person loses their sense of what is real and true for them. This has an extremely destructive impact on a person's sense of self and their ability to act.

Religious

Religious abuse describes the ways in which one person or group coerces another into following a particular set of religious beliefs or practices.

Honour

Honour abuse is a cohesive, often criminal, attack to protect or defend the 'honour' of a family or community. It is often, if not always, motivated by the collective shame of the community and the individual shame of the perpetrator. If a family member or community leader thinks someone has shamed or embarrassed them by behaving in a certain way – being gay, engaging in a relationship outside the community, having sex before marriage, being disabled – they may punish that person for breaking their 'honour' code.

Domestic abuse

Domestic abuse consists of different forms of abuse that take place in the context of the home, between caregivers and the people they care for or between family members or partners. Domestic abuse is often hidden from others, and it can be particularly difficult to disclose or to ask for help with. It can include

- Physical abuse
- Psychological abuse
- Financial abuse
- Sexual abuse
- Neglect
- Any combination of the above

Elder abuse

Elder abuse is similar to domestic abuse and targets older people. It can take place at home or in a care setting. Perpetrators are often known to the victim and can be relatives, neighbours, or care home staff or volunteers. As with other forms of abuse, it can range from physical or sexual abuse to financial exploitation.

Intimate partner violence

Intimate partner violence is abuse perpetrated by an intimate partner. It can be experienced as physical or psychological abuse, controlling behaviour, rape, or sexual abuse and/or stalking. Anyone can be a victim of this type of abuse.

County lines and exploitation

County lines is a term used in the UK to describe a type of criminal exploitation in which criminal organisations coerce or force children and young people to store drugs, money, or weapons and move them to suburban areas or areas outside of large urban environments. Perpetrators can groom children and young people to take part in this risky behaviour, often exposing them to other forms of abuse or crime, such as sexual abuse, knife crime, human trafficking, etc. County lines distances the perpetrators from the criminal act and leaves the children with the risk of carrying out the illegal activity.

Modern slavery

Modern slavery is the illegal exploitation of someone for either personal or commercial gain. It can include many types of abuse, including sexual exploitation, domestic servitude, forced labour, organ harvesting, or criminal exploitation. Victims can be tricked or threatened into work and may feel unable to leave or report the crime due to fear or intimidation. Often, victims of modern slavery are trafficked into the UK, though victims of modern slavery who are from the UK tend to have been exploited from a pre-existing position of vulnerability.

State-sanctioned abuse

State-sanctioned abuse covers all abuse that is either caused directly by the government or upheld through institutional bias or discrimination. Examples include racial profiling and acts of violence towards vulnerable people by police. It can also include policies that negatively target certain groups, such as policies that aim to 'catch out' disabled people or those in poverty and prevent them from accessing the support or benefits they need.

Stalking

Stalking can often be mistaken for harassment or repeated annoying behaviour, but it's more aggressive and serious in reality. A stalker is obsessed with the person they're targeting. Stalkers can be ex-partners, friends, or strangers, and stalking can take place in person or online. The four warning signs of stalking are behaviour that is experienced as

- **F**ixated
- **O**bsessive
- **U**nwanted
- **R**epeated

Spiking

Spiking is giving someone alcohol or drugs without them consenting. It can be done by putting alcohol or drugs in their drink, vape, or in a needle. Doing this makes the victim vulnerable, tired, unconscious, or unable to function normally. It makes someone vulnerable to robbery or sexual abuse or rape.

Types of sexual abuse

Sexual abuse is inflicting sexual contact upon a person against their will or engaging in sexual contact with a person who is unable to legally consent due to age or mental or physical incapacity. Sexual abuse is rarely, if ever, about desire or sexuality; rather, it is about control, exploitation, and power. Different types of sexual abuse are listed below.

Childhood sexual abuse

Childhood sexual abuse is abuse that happens to a child. It can be perpetrated by an adult or a similarly aged child. It often happens in the home or institutions that hold authority within communities, like schools, boarding schools, sports or youth clubs, or religious institutions (although it is not exclusive to these places).

Adolescent sexual abuse

Abuse that happens to teenagers is often grouped as the same as abuse experienced by children. However, I want to distinguish adolescence as separate from childhood for a few reasons. Adolescence is a unique time during which a person can face many developmental changes and challenges, and the speed of the brain and body's development during this period is comparable to that seen in a toddler. Adolescence is also a time that can affect the rest of a person's life. Most harmful health behaviours, such as smoking, start during this time, and three-quarters of serious mental health issues start before the age of 24. Despite this, teenagers are constantly overlooked in healthcare settings, meaning a lot of traumatised young people fall through the cracks and are missed. Teens who are abused often face specific stigma. Girls can be called slutty or accused of 'asking for it', whereas boys are called 'lucky'. Adolescents of all genders face assumptions that they know what they are doing, can consent, or are in some way to blame for abuse. This is never the case. Teenagers are just as vulnerable as children to attacks or coercion by people who hold power over them.

People who were abused as children or teenagers can find themselves in the painful position of looking back at their abuse with complicated feelings, especially if the abuser was someone close to them. At this vulnerable age, we can want the attention of adults, particularly if we grow up in unstable environments or face neglect. Children and teenagers who experience sexual abuse can be manipulated into silence or seeking out the abuse from their abusers. This is called *grooming*, and it is damaging because feelings of closeness to an abuser can be powerful and stay with us into adulthood. Teenagers are often assumed to be mature enough to consent to sex, a viewpoint that ignores the vulnerability of this life stage. It's also a form of adultification. As Davis and March explain,

> The concept of adultification is when notions of innocence and vulnerability are not afforded to certain children. This is determined by people and institutions who hold power over them. When adultification occurs outside of the home it is always founded within discrimination and bias.
>
> There are various definitions of adultification, all related to a child's personal characteristics, socio-economic influences and/or lived experiences. Regardless of the context in which adultification takes place, the impact results in children's rights being either diminished or not upheld.[10]

Black children and teenagers are particularly vulnerable to adultification. This often happens when they interact with statutory organisations, such as those within the care, healthcare, education, and justice systems.

Young people who physically or behaviourally mature quicker than their peers also face adultification. A defence perpetrators use is 'they were mature for their age', again ignoring the victim's vulnerability. Teenagers can be good at appearing mature; it's an important life stage, like trying on adulting before becoming an adult. It is not maturity built on emotional, physical, social, and intellectual ground that adult maturity is built on. Teenagers who act mature are doing just that: acting. Their emotional maturity does not develop into adulthood until much later in life.

Intrafamilial sexual abuse (or incest)

Intrafamilial abuse is abuse of a child or adolescent within the family environment. The perpetrator may be related to the survivor or may be a close friend of the family. This type of abuse often goes undisclosed for many years due to how shameful it can feel. It is common that people who survive this have survived other abuses, such as physical abuse or emotional neglect.

Child-on-child sexual abuse

Child-on-child sexual abuse can be defined as sexual activity between children that happens without consent or equality due to differences in mental or physical capacity or age. It can result from coercion and is often a result of a power difference between children. It is often unreported or dismissed by adults, viewed as natural experimentation between children.

In this situation both children need help. The child who has been abused needs appropriate and professional support, and the child who engaged in the abuse or harmful sexual behaviour needs support as such behaviour is often an indicator of harm or vulnerability in the perpetrating child's life.

Sibling sexual abuse

Sexual abuse between siblings is a common form of intrafamilial and child-on-child sexual abuse. It's common for social workers or protection agencies to encounter it. Children often develop sexual behaviours as a natural part of growing up, acting them out on siblings or cousins due to their proximity and similar ages.

Professionals need to be on the lookout for signs that this natural development stage could become harmful in some way. Commonly, social workers or child psychologists may try and spot

- Behaviour that upsets other children involved
- Behaviour that happens often or seems compulsive
- Behaviour that forces other children to engage, either through aggression or pressure
- Behaviour that is directed towards adults, rather than peers or members of a child's own age group (this can also include interest towards children with a significant age difference)
- Behaviour that affects other activities, such as clubs, school or hobbies
- Use of pornography, graphic or explicit images (this can include sending and receiving images or videos via mobile phones or tablets).

Survivors can have mixed feelings about this type of abuse and perpetrator, because they were both children, are related, and often still have a relationship. Each case comes with its own nuance, but if you feel uncomfortable or that what happened crossed a boundary, it is likely that some imbalance of power led to a lack of consent, either given or understood.

It can take time to figure out how you feel about this, but remember, the way *you* feel is important. Other people don't get to dictate what was abusive or harmful.

Non-contact sexual abuse

Non-contact abuse occurs when a child is sexually abused without physical contact with the abuser. This can happen in person, online, or over phone messaging services. It can include sharing pornography with a child or coercing them into sharing explicit photos of themselves, making videos of themselves masturbating, or having sexually explicit conversations. It can also include the abuser exposing or flashing themselves or forcing the child to do the same.

Online sexual abuse

Online sexual abuse predominately effects children or young people and occurs when a person is coerced, groomed, or tricked into sexual activities over the internet. This can include actively engaging in online sexual activity via video chat rooms or using audio or typed communication. It is often overlooked in books and resources on sexual abuse. Despite this, online sexual abuse is not a new problem but one that is constantly changing and evolving with technology.

Self-generated online sexual abuse

Self-generated online sexual abuse occurs when sexual content is created by a child using a camera phone or webcam and is shared online via different platforms. This can include material initially created by a child victim of online abuse that is then shared. Children may livestream (filming in real time) without knowing they are being recorded for later distribution by the abuser. Children and young people may also create sexual material that they share with an abuser, who then distributes it without their knowledge. Many children and young people are unaware that the person they are talking to online is not a 'friend' but someone coercing them for sexual content to be shared later.

Children and young people from specific communities or identities may be especially vulnerable to this type of abuse. This is due partly to their unique vulnerabilities and also to the ways that different young people use the internet. The Internet Watch Foundation has found that young people with special educational needs and disabilities (SEND) can be particularly vulnerable:

- A child with complex needs may be less likely to understand or recognise the signs of online sexual abuse.
- A lack of awareness may result from poorer access to information regarding online harms.
- Some SEND children may interpret things literally or struggle to understand more abstract concepts, such as why an adult might pretend to be a child online.
- Children with reduced emotional processing skills may be more vulnerable to attention from others, including adults looking to groom them online.
- In addition, if a child struggles with communicating their feelings or needs, they may find it harder to disclose experiences that make them feel uncomfortable.[11]

LGBTQIA+ young people can struggle to find community in their school or college, and the internet can offer valuable space for them to meet others from similar backgrounds. According to a 2017 Stonewall report, 96 per cent of young people say the internet has helped them to understand more about their sexual orientation and/or gender identity. However, 45 per cent have received or sent sexual, naked or semi-naked material to a person they were talking to online and one in five LGBTQIA+ youth under 18 has used an 18+ dating app such as Tinder, Grindr or Her. This environment can make them more vulnerable to perpetrators online.

Sextortion

In August 2024, *The Guardian* newspaper[12] investigated sextortion guides and manuals found on social media platforms like TikTok and YouTube. These are instructional videos or written manuals detailing how to trick teenagers into sending nude or sexual material of themselves to then extort money from them under the threat of releasing the sexual material. This abusive violation can be extremely emotionally damaging as it involves emotional manipulation, sexual abuse and extortion.

Cyberflashing

Cyberflashing is a relatively new term that describes sending unsolicited nude images to someone via a dating app, chat platform, AirDrop, Bluetooth, email, or some other digital device. It has been a crime in Scotland since 2010 and became a crime in England in 2022 as part of the Online Safety Act. The first UK prison sentence for cyberflashing occurred in March 2024, when a man in the UK was sentenced to 66 weeks in prison after he sent unsolicited photos of his erect penis on 9 February 2024 to a 15-year-old girl and a woman via the Whatsapp and iMessage apps.

Adulthood sexual abuse

Abuse that happens in adulthood can be difficult for men to come to terms with. Social stigma can be really damaging. 'Why didn't you fight them off?' is often something that men hear from police, doctors, nurses, even partners and spouses, when disclosing. A big part of that stigma is the idea that sexual abuse or rape can't happen to men at all. Men who experience abuse in adulthood are one of the least talked about and most marginalised groups of sexual abuse survivors. Men can be vulnerable to assault from any gender, including women, and they can be abused in any context: in relationships, during attacks on a night out, or due to pressure or coercion resulting from power imbalances.

Stealthing

Stealthing is the practice of non-consensually removing a condom during penetrative sex. It is a violation of the agreed terms of sexual consent (ie, using condoms) and exposes people to sexually transmitted diseases or unwanted pregnancies. In the United States, California became the first state to make stealthing illegal, in 2021, though it is only a civil offence (meaning survivors are only able to sue the perpetrator, rather than bring them to criminal court). In England and Wales, the practice is considered rape and carries the potential for a lifetime prison sentence. While *stealthing* is a slang word, the term the English and Welsh legal system uses for it is rape.

Revenge porn

Revenge porn has only been illegal in the UK since 2015, under the Criminal Justice and Courts ACT 2015. Under this law, distributing private intimate, sexual, naked, or semi-naked images of someone without their consent and with the intent to cause distress or embarrassment is a crime, as is threatening to do so. In some cases, images are shared along with the victim's personal information, such as their full name, address, contact details, or social media accounts.

This offence is often thought of as an online abuse, but the 2015 law also covers physically showing images of a person, either in person, on a phone, or via printed material.

Sex trafficking

Human sex trafficking is a form of modern slavery in which the victim is forced into sexual acts with paying perpetrators. Violence, manipulation, coercion, and fraud are all used to recruit and control a vulnerable person. Trafficked people may depend on their traffickers financially (debt bondage) or emotionally. Trafficking effects people of all ages and genders; however, the most vulnerable people are refugees or migrant workers, people with disabilities, survivors of past trauma, or young people who have been in the care system.

A note on language

Abuse, assault, trauma, rape

According to the Sexual Offences Act 2003, '[t]he legal definition of rape is when a person intentionally penetrates another's vagina, anus or mouth with a penis, without the other person's consent', whereas '[a]ssault by penetration is when a person penetrates another person's vagina or anus with any part of the body other than a penis, or by using an object, without the person's consent'.[13]

For survivors of all genders, these classifications can be reductive and unhelpful in defining their experience and in their recovery. Each survivor will find their own language that fits their own experience. The terms *sexual abuse, sexual assault, rape,* and *sexual trauma* all carry different meanings for different people. For some, the word *assault* feels sudden, violent and almost random, whereas *abuse* is relational, cohesive, secretive. *Trauma* can be a strong word; for some, this will feel appropriate, while others may find it difficult to feel their abuse was serious enough to use strong words about it. In this book, I use these words interchangeably to speak to as many people's experiences as possible.

Sexual minorities: Queer or LGBTQIA+?

In this intersectional book, I discuss multiple different groups of men, including members of sexual minority groups. To refer to this community, I use the term *LGBTQIA+* rather than the term *queer*. *Queer*, once a slur for gay people, is increasingly used as an identifier for members of sexual minority groups. It also describes various political, activist, and academic frameworks concerned with members of sexual minority groups and social/political change. However, for some, the word still carries negative and sometimes traumatic associations. Additionally, in some parts of the world, it remains a slur. I celebrate the transformation of the word from a slur to a word associated with social change, but I want to acknowledge that it does not yet carry that meaning for everyone, and thus, I have not used it in this book.

Men or male?

I will use the word 'men' and 'male' interchangeably throughout the text where appropriate. For many reading this book, this distinction won't matter. However, for some, particularly those questioning their gender, the difference between male, as in 'sex', and men, as in 'gender', may be important and is rarely acknowledged in similar literature. All to say, if you identify as male, or masculinity shapes your experience of the abuse, this space is for you.

You've done it! You've made it to the end of the introduction. Much like you would if you were finishing the first session of a recovery group, you now have a sense of what is to come. From here on, each chapter will reflect on a different theme commonly experienced by male survivors. Go at your own pace, take notes, take tea breaks, and take care of yourself. This is your journey, and I am honoured and humbled to share some of it with you.

Blank Pages

Each chapter ends with a blank page. They are there for you to use. There is no right or wrong way to use them. You could consider:

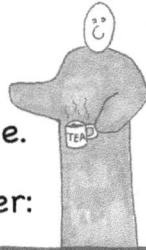

Write down interesting facts or observations

you find in the book,

Things you might want to research or look up later

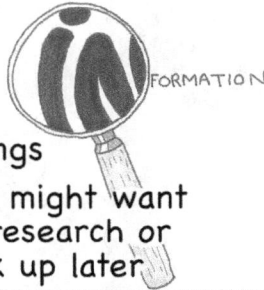

FORMATION

Questions that come up you might want to ask a friend, ally or therapist.

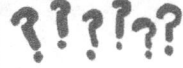

Draw or doodle to help you

process feelings or emotions

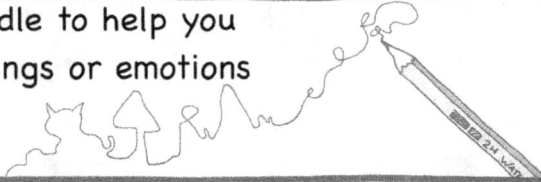

If you're not sure how to start, maybe take a look at the emotions wheel at the back of this book. Pick a few emotions you feel and make a note of them in this blank space. Then, next time you pick up this book, see if your emotions have changed and ask yourself, what has caused a change in these emotions?

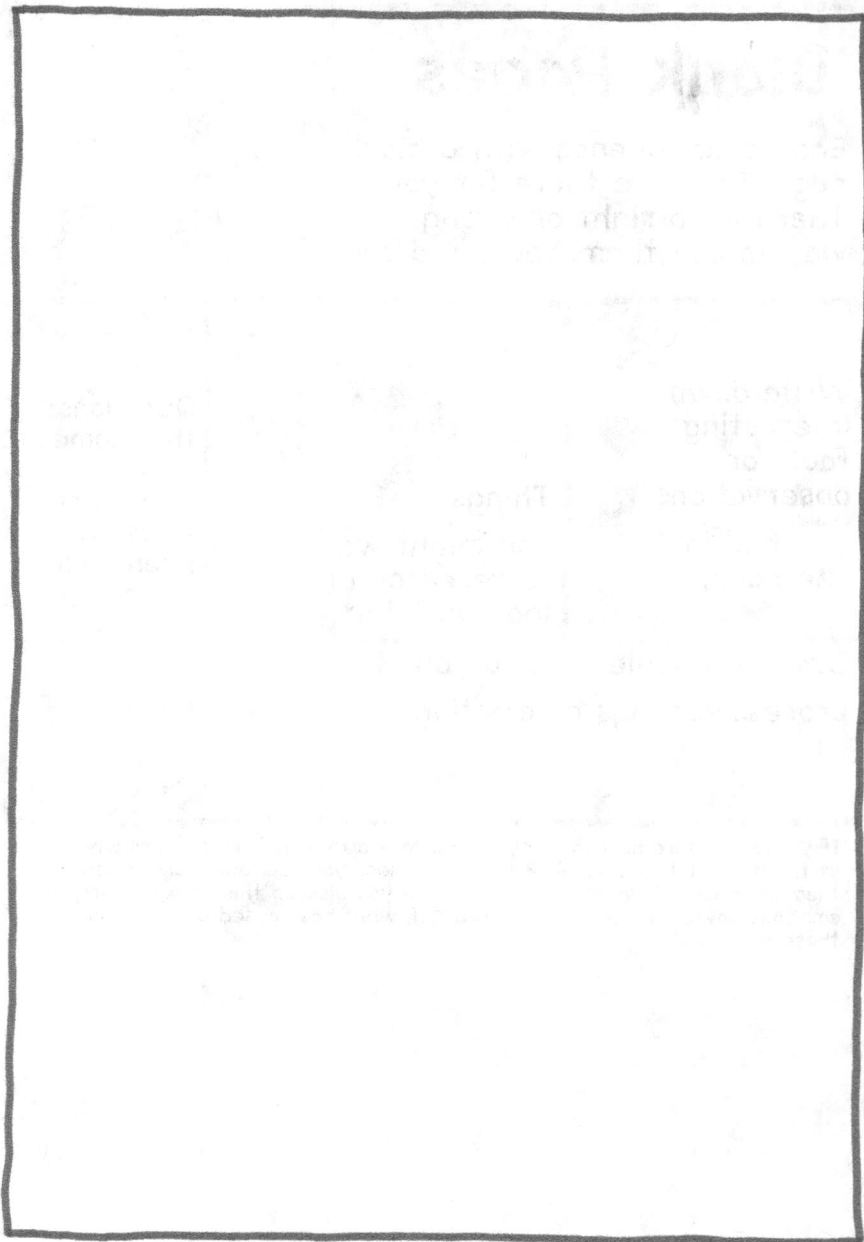

For A4 and printable versions of this worksheet, visit www.jeremysachs.com

Notes

1 'William James: Quotes: Quotable quote', Goodreads. https://www.goodreads.com/quo tes/837455-we-are-like-islands-in-the-sea-separate-on-the, accessed 20 February 2025.
2 World Health Organization, 'Men's health', WHO Regional Office for Europe, last updated 16 September 2018. https://www.who.int/europe/news-room/fact-sheets/item/men-s-health, accessed 2 August 2024.
3 'Key data: mortality', Men's Health Forum, January 2017. www.menshealthforum.org.uk/key-data-mortality, accessed 28 May 2024.
4 'Key data: Understanding health and access to services', Men's Health Forum, 2024. www.menshealthforum.org.uk/key-data-understanding-health-and-access-services, accessed 28 May 2024.
5 David A. Ramsay and Sarah Bunn, 'POST: Men's health', UK Parliament, 12 December 2023. https://researchbriefings.files.parliament.uk/documents/POST-PB-0056/POST-PB-0056.pdf, accessed 28 May 2024.
6 'Suicides in England and Wales: 2022 registrations', Office for National Statistics, 19 December 2023. www.ons.gov.uk/peoplepopulationandcommunity/birthsdeathsandma rriages/deaths/bulletins/suicidesintheunitedkingdom/2022registrations, accessed 28 May 2024.
7 'Probable suicides in Scotland: 2022 report', National Records of Scotland, 5 September 2023. www.nrscotland.gov.uk/files/statistics/probable-suicides/2022/suicides-22-rep ort.pdf, accessed 28 May 2024.
8 'Kimberlé Crenshaw on intersectionality, more than two decades later', Columbia Law School, 8 June 2017. www.law.columbia.edu/news/archive/kimberle-crenshaw-inters ectionality-more-two-decades-later, accessed 28 May 2024.
9 Kimberlé Crenshaw, 'The urgency of intersectionality', TED, October 2016. www. ted.com/talks/kimberle_crenshaw_the_urgency_of_intersectionality?language=en, accessed 28 May 2024.
10 Jahnine Davis and Nicholas Marsh, 'The Myth of the Universal Child', in *Safeguarding Young People: Risk, Rights, Relationships and Resilience*, ed. D. Holmes (London: Jessica Kingsley Publishers, 2022), 111–128.
11 'Make sure your home doesn't have an open door to child sexual abusers', Internet Watch Foundation, 2024. https://talk.iwf.org.uk, accessed 28 May 2024.
12 Samuel Osborne, 'Video "Sextortion Guides" and Manuals Found on TikTok and YouTube.' *The Guardian*, 22 August 2024. https://www.theguardian.com/uk-news/arti cle/2024/aug/22/video-sextortion-guides-and-manuals-found-on-tiktok-and-youtube.
13 'What is rape and sexual assault?', Metropolitan Police, 2024. www.met.police.uk/adv ice/advice-and-information/rsa/rape-and-sexual-assault/what-is-rape-and-sexual-assa ult/#:~:text=The%20legal%20definition%20of%20rape,without%20the%20other%20 person's%20consent, accessed 10 July 2024.

Chapter 2

What we mean when we say 'trauma'

Chapter Contents

Managing my trauma

I struggle with anxiety, nightmares, and constantly feeling on edge. Sometimes I find myself dissociating or having panic attacks out of the blue. Which is mad to swing between the two, not really knowing which way I'll go. I don't know if that's the trauma or if I get that from my mum. I don't like admitting it, but she did the same when we were kids. I've found that smoking weed helps; it softens the hard edges. It's also something I can enjoy doing with my pals – probably the only good relationships I have in my life. I'd rather go to the GP to get meds, but that feels stressful and like they would ask me lots of questions I don't want to answer. That's where my therapy is at right now, working up to making an appointment. But also, the weed kills my dreams, so that's a good side effect for now.

I only talked about my abuse for the first time eight months ago because I need to sort my life out. I want to go back to college and get into IT, but to do that I need to sort out how the abuse has impacted me and my relationships. I need to be able to stick to things and follow through without self-sabotaging or getting overwhelmed.

Trying to heal from the abuse is hard because you're doing it at the same time as trying to build a life, and you're like, *This would be easier if I could stop the trauma for just a second, but they all get tangled up with each other and I don't know what's the trauma and what's just me, where does it stop and I begin?* I know it doesn't work like that, but you get so angry thinking how

DOI: 10.4324/9781003423331-2

the abuse sets you back and keeps stopping you moving forward. Despite that, I will enrol in college, just to know that the abuse hasn't beaten me. I don't want it to control my life; I want to be in the driving seat for once.

Anonymous, 24 years old, from Clydebank, Scotland

2.1   Trauma

In 2015, I was working for a charity in North London. Our road was shared by lots of other charities of all sizes, from international non-governmental organisations (NGOs) to small, localised outfits with two members of staff. This was the first time I remember hearing the term *'trauma informed'*. Suddenly it was everywhere. Charity workers were being encouraged to do trauma-informed training and charities were changing mission statements to include a 'trauma focus' to be more eligible for highly competitive funding. In their personal lives, people had a new term to describe painful experiences in childhood. *Trauma* had become the buzzword of the moment. Unlike most buzzwords, however, it has endured. The word *trauma* is still commonly used in the charity sector, in the therapy room, and among individuals describing their experiences. Some of this may be 'concept creep', a phenomenon where the meanings of psychological terms such as *trauma*, as well as diagnostic terms such as *OCD* and *post-traumatic stress disorder (PTSD)*, change because more people use them in everyday language.[1] The words *creep* from the clinical meaning to a more colloquial, everyday meaning. While this gets criticised, I don't mind it because it feels like people have more access to psychological language than ever before. Even the complexities of trauma are more accessible, from books, podcasts, and YouTube videos to wellbeing influencers on social media. There are lots of new sources of information to help us make sense of our own experiences.

So where does that leave this chapter? How can it add to the growing public discussions about trauma and be useful to survivors? In an attempt to answer this question, the chapter will summarise the Defence Cascade – how our brains respond in order to keep us safe when we experience a sexual abuse. We will also look at how sexual trauma may impact people differently, depending on identity, support networks, and past experiences. Lastly, I've pulled together a brief, contemporary look at where male survivors are situated within society now and how recent events might impact their ability to access support. The next chapter will look at the lasting legacy of trauma and different symptoms that might impact survivors long after abuse, as well as suggestions on how to talk about trauma using language that feels right to us.

At the end of this chapter, as with most chapters in this book, you'll find further resources and signposting you might want to investigate to deepen your knowledge about the themes introduced in this chapter.

What is trauma?

Trauma isn't an event or experience that happens to you. It is your mind and body's response to that event or experience. As Dr Gabor Maté, addiction expert, says, trauma 'is not what happens to you; it is what happens inside you as a result of what happens to you'.[2]

Abuse creates strong responses in our bodies and minds, and for some these responses get stuck. Many years after our abuse, we can still have flashbacks and nightmares that leave us terrified. Smells can bring on panic attacks and the historical abuse we survived feels like it's happening all over again.

Some men manage to repress and forget their abuse, leading a 'normal' life until one day, something happens that reminds them of the abuse, and memories come flooding back, drowning them in trauma responses, panic and fear. Whether you have been living with the memories of abuse or whether you have recently had abuse memories resurface, here is a list of common experiences men have told me activate their trauma responses:

- You undergo an invasive medical procedure, such as a dentist appointment or operation.
- A child in your life reaches the same age you were when abused.
- A sexual encounter goes wrong, or you feel high levels of stress around sex.
- Another trauma happens, such as a car crash, and shakes loose historical trauma.
- A parent or significant person from your childhood dies.
- A current sexual assault suddenly reminds you of earlier abuses.
- You experience high stress at home or at work.
- Sensory memories come back; smells, songs, films or TV shows unlock past memories.
- You undergo certain types of therapy or spend time reflecting on your past.
- You hear about other people's experience of sexual trauma, either in person or through TV shows.

This is not an exhaustive list, but it gives you an idea of how traumatic memories can be activated. When this happens, it can leave survivors feeling all sorts of different ways. We all experience traumatic symptoms differently. Again, the list below is not exhaustive, but you might recognise some of these symptoms from your experience:

- Having flashbacks, bad dreams or poor sleep
- Experiencing physical aches, pains, or poor physical health
- Swinging between heightened emotional states and feeling nothing at all
- Experiencing emotional responses disproportionate to the situation
- Zoning out, feeling numb, or getting sleepy in conflict or stress
- Experiencing depression and anxiety

- Living with a mental health diagnosis such as a personality disorder, complex Post-Traumatic Stress Disorder (cPTSD), or psychosis
- Becoming overly attached to people very quickly
- Struggling to attach to anyone
- Swinging wildly between feeling understood by someone and feeling distant, unseen, or resentful towards them

The experience of trauma can extend beyond thoughts and feelings into behaviour. Much of this behaviour is in some way designed to manage the traumatic feelings, even if the behaviour is detrimental to our health. These are some health behaviours often associated with trauma:

- Addictions
- Unhealthy work patterns
- Struggling to look after your health (eating healthy food or doing physical activity)
- Overdependence on wellness and fitness
- Sexual issues (complete disinterest in sex or constantly seeking out sex/masturbation)
- Acting with anger or frustration, often punishing people around you or taking it out on yourself
- Difficulty maintaining boundaries in friends
- Self-sabotaging relationships
- Being attracted to other abusive people
- Constantly minimising mental health issues by avoiding getting help because it feels like no one could understand or you're not worth help

It's important to bear in mind any one of these behaviours alone is not a stand-alone indicator of trauma. Many people engage in these behaviours and have not experienced something traumatic. We can't use them to diagnose abuse. However, they are common among those of us living with the impact of sexual trauma. Self-medicating with drugs or alcohol or soothing and distracting with work, sex, or food can be lifesaving strategies for some survivors seeking to either regulate emotions, numb pain or create a feeling of euphoria and aliveness (as the author of the testimony in this chapter demonstrates, by smoking marijuana).[3]

The reason trauma can have such a dramatic effect on us long after the danger has passed is that it taps into a primal emotional state. Hard-wired into all of us are defence responses that have been present since the beginning of humanity. When these defence responses are activated, they can take over quickly, and this can be overwhelming or beyond our control. What activates defence responses can be varied and unpredictable. What might be traumatic for one person may not be for another. War, immigration, natural disasters, witnessing or being the victim of violence, complex bereavement, sudden life-threatening accidents, and of course, sexual abuse: these are all deeply disturbing, but may not feel traumatising to everyone.

You may have heard of the fight, flight, or freeze response, in which a victim attempts to fight off an aggressor, run away or freeze during a traumatic event. This response is part of what happens in the brain, but it isn't our entire response to trauma. What we are increasingly learning is that the fight, flight, or freeze response isn't necessarily the brain automatically choosing one of these options out of the blue. Rather, it is part of a process that the body and brain go through together. This can be interesting for male survivors to hear, because so often they are asked (or ask themselves), 'Why didn't you fight back?', as if they had a choice. It can be alarming to think that we chose to freeze and simply accept our fates. Culturally, not 'fighting back' contradicts society's expectations of us (see Chapter 4, page 62). The truth is, we simply could not have fought back. We would have had to fight off not only a perpetrator who was in a position of power over us, but also millennia of evolutionary growth designed to minimise the physical and mental damage that a trauma can cause. This process is called *the Defence Cascade*.

Before I go into detail on the Defence Cascade, I want to invite you to check in with yourself. I've found survivors can be surprised at how emotional they get learning about this. The offer of information, especially that which is evidence-based and often shared with the intention of supporting a person's understanding of their mental health, is called psychoeducation. Psychoeducation can lend itself to a more clinical, or detached, tone while we are simultaneously being taken back to some of the most painful experiences we have survived. This can be jarring and upsetting. Make sure you're in a comfortable, safe space when reading. Allow yourself tea breaks, a stretch, or to grab something that makes you feel comfortable.

The Defence Cascade

The Defence Cascade[4] is a set of responses to threats that has been studied in humans and animals. It is an instinctual 'continuum of innate, hard-wired, automatically activated defensive behaviours in response to threats'[5] that cascades through different defence stages. There are various models of Defence Cascade, but this version adapted from the Harvard Review of Psychiatry is one I find useful:

1. **Arousal.** *Arousal* is a word often associated with the erotic or sexual, but this definition is broader. It describes a state high alertness, in which we have sensed a threat or a highly stressful situation. The heartbeat becomes louder and faster, the mouth dries, stress hormones start generating, and sweat is generated regardless of heat. In this stage, we are ready to act and we either cascade to the second stage (*fight or flight*) or, far more commonly for sexual abuse survivors, to the third or fourth stages (*freeze* or *tonic immobility*).
2. **Fight or flight.** Fight or flight is generally a common response to threats or stress. You may have seen this in children who, when traumatised or struggling to emotionally regulate, will run away or fly into a rage. In adults, we see this

response often in those living with complex PTSD. They may become confrontational, violent, or go to lengths to escape from situations. The response is less common during sexual abuse. It's extremely rare to hear of people responding to the abuse itself with fight or flight. By nature, sexual abuse often involves not just an abuse of body but an abuse of power too. The mind is unlikely to cascade to fight or flight if it decides it's unlikely to be effective and, in some cases, might make the situation potentially more dangerous.

3. **Freeze.** Freezing is normally a very brief stage that can last only a few seconds as we cascade through the different stages. It typically occurs at the beginning of a threat and can be experienced as similar to the first stage, arousal. Unlike arousal, however, there can be a slowing of the heart rate. We are alert, tense and still. We still have a cognitive understanding of what is going on around us. Interestingly, for those who are exposed to multiple threats throughout their lives, there is evidence that our bodies can become primed for a freeze response, ready to freeze in the face of threat.[6]

4. **Tonic immobility.** Tonic immobility occurs across many different species. In addition to humans, it is seen in sharks, possums (who 'play dead' better than anyone!), snakes, beetles, ducks... the list goes on. Be they mammal, vertebrate, invertebrate, bird, or reptile, most species will have this threat defence. It's also very common during a sexual assault. This defence can show up as an inability to move, call for help, or feel pain, as well as coldness and dissociative experiences such as emotional numbing or out of body experiences. This stage of the cascade is often confused with the freeze response. However, unlike freeze, it can be completely disabling: our bodies, like possums, are playing dead, and it's difficult to respond to our surroundings or what is happening. In addition to sexual abuse survivors, accounts of tonic immobility are common in traumatised soldiers, animal attack victims. and car or plan crash survivors.

5. **Collapsed immobility.** This defence was added to the Defence Cascade relatively recently, in 2004.[7] It is similar to tonic immobility, but in addition to 'playing dead', our muscles lose the ability to hold us, and we experience partial or complete lack of consciousness. This can be described as the most extreme defence in the Defence Cascade. Some have conceptualised it as preparing for death, as our body and mind have gone numb, and we can no longer feel pain.

6. **Quiescent immobility.** Once a danger has passed and we are able to acknowledge that we have survived and feel relatively safe, our body and mind need to recover. Every part of us has been pushed to its limits while cascading through these threat responses. For many of us, the body and its systems have never experienced anything this stressful before. Our heart has potentially sped up and slowed, our senses have become hyper-aroused to our environment and then numbed, our brains have produced huge amounts of stress hormones, our pain receptors have dulled, and our muscles have frozen and then collapsed. I would argue that there is nothing in our everyday lives that can prepare our

whole body for such an assault. Quiescent immobility is easily spotted in animals that have near-death experiences. Imagine a deer that escapes a big cat attack. The deer stands still, breathes, maybe shakes. Its bodily systems are taking time to recover. While this post-threat recuperation has been observed in animals, there is less post-assault research in humans.

I hope that reading this helps you to understand that when we experience something as disturbing and complicated as sexual abuse, our mind and body need to deploy some extreme defences. Survivors, particularly male survivors, face disbelief and stigma: 'Why didn't you fight back or call for help?' Or the alternative, 'Why did you just let it happen?' It can be easy for men to internalise these questions and blame themselves, when in reality, their body and mind were doing the best they could to survive.

While running group therapy, I might condense these trauma responses to be more accessible by breaking them down into the 'Five F's': **Fight, Flight, Freeze, Flop,** and **Friend:**

- **Fight.** Fight is an unlikely defence in cases of sexual abuse. It occurs when a victim attempts to fight off a threat. It's most common in distressed children or those who live with long-term traumatic stress disorders like cPTSD. Importantly, children and those with traumatic stress disorders are also unlikely to fight if they experience sexual abuse.
- **Flight.** Flight is also an unlikely response to sexual abuse. It occurs when a victim attempts to flee a threat. It is an unlikely option due to its low probability of success and the potential for further harm if caught or prevented from fleeing.
- **Freeze.** Within the Defence Cascade, freeze is the tonic immobility defence. This is a highly likely response. When a victim freezes, their muscles tense, and they feel paralysed. If an attack occurs over a prolonged period of time, it is likely that the freeze then develops into flop.
- **Flop.** In the Defence Cascade, flop is the collapsed immobility defence that can involve passing out or loss of consciousness. Like freeze, flop is a common response to sexual abuse. If you struggle to remember details of your assault, as well as the hours before or after, it could be because you experienced freeze or flop, both of which compromise your ability to create and retain memories.
- **Friend (sometimes called Fawn).** This response typically happens on either side of the freeze or flop response. It occurs when a victim calls out for help, hoping to enlist support from a bystander or attempts to appease an attacker to avoid harm or further harm.

However, for survivors, the friend response can have an alternative meaning outside of a trauma response. I have heard survivors talk about being in longstanding relationships with an abuser. They try to cultivate a 'friendship' with the abuser to avoid future abuse. This is not unusual in cases of domestic abuse, child abuse, or scenarios where a survivor has been imprisoned by a perpetrator for a prolonged time. When living with an abusive person, survivors often do everything they can to control their environment and the abusive person in order to reduce the chances that they will become abusive. Abuse victims are doing constant 'risk assessments' to determine if a situation may lead to abuse. In this way, they are 'friending' the abuser in an attempt to control their behaviour and hopefully avoid experiencing abuse. This can include, in some cases, agreeing to sex. It is really important to acknowledge that this is not consenting to sex. Saying 'yes' to sex or sexual contact in order to prevent escalating abuse or avoid confrontation is not consenting to sex; it is an instinctive and sophisticated survival mechanism.

This form of friending may be familiar to gay, trans, or nonbinary people living with homophobic and abusive family members or to disabled or older men relying on abusive partners for care. Friending someone abusive, for many survivors, is an attempt to gain power in a dynamic where we find ourselves powerless.

2.2   Not all sexual abuse is traumatic

If you're reading this chapter and thinking to yourself, *Neither the Defence Cascade nor the Five F's apply to how I feel*, you may not have experienced a clinical version of trauma. This does not mean the abuse was not deeply disturbing, stressful, or frightening – simply that your brain did not rely on the Defence Cascade. Alternatively, you might have cycled through the Defence Cascade and, after the abuse, been able to process it well enough not to cause lasting pain. Or maybe you were able to bury trauma symptoms away for decades. Not all people respond to sexual abuse in the same way, and as such, each person's experience needs to be viewed individually. This can feel particularly true for men, who often have their experience minimised, homogenised, or diminished.

Lots of things can factor into how we respond to sexual abuse, including the presence of contextual protective or exacerbating factors:

Contextual protective factors. These are positive circumstances that allow a person to process and recover from trauma. They can be practical things like access to healthcare – both living somewhere with specialised services or therapy and being able to travel to and afford such services. Other protective circumstances can include a lack of previous stressful or traumatic experiences prior to the sexual abuse or having family or friends that are open to talking about the abuse without risk of disbelief or further complicating the situation.

Exacerbating factors. These are negative circumstances that can make recovering from sexual abuse more challenging. Examples include health inequalities, such as a lack of a specialised services or barriers to accessing them, including poor public transport, disability or lack of finances. A history of negative experiences with healthcare organisations can also create barriers. This can include personal experiences, like previous types of abuse from healthcare or belonging to a community that has been disproportionally let down or harmed by healthcare services. In some cases, men don't seek out support because of societal expectations on them. Many men do not want to waste a doctor's time or do not reveal the severity of their pain. Others simply feel they ought to be able to deal with it by themselves. Additional exacerbating factors can include complicated relationships with family, growing up around further abuses, poverty, or stressful environments.

When I think about protective and exacerbating factors, I conceptualise them into two different statements:

- **Protective:** I have gone through something that brought me closer to others.
- **Exacerbating:** I have gone through something that makes me feel isolated and alone.

This comes back to intersectionality. A survivor's identity and circumstances will play a role in their vulnerability to, experience of, and recovery from trauma.[8] Those who belong to a minority group or who find themselves powerless in some way might have a greater struggle in recovery. On top of this, some mental health services or charities that support survivors do not take culture and identity into account. Services are often siloed, focusing on trauma systems but missing the context of how traumas are experienced. The danger with this is that parts of each individual's trauma, pain and story are missed, which then becomes a missed opportunity to support healing.

I've found when speaking to many men that certain behaviours, beliefs, or even traumas are passed down to them from their parents. These can be separate from sexual abuse but can make it hard for men to heal from sexual abuse they encounter. For these men, it can help to consider intergenerational trauma: trauma experienced by older generations in our family or community that affects us today. We can inherit the trauma of our parents, grandparents or elders around us.

Intergenerational trauma

We inherit lots from our parents. Most obviously, we inherit how we look: eye colour, hair texture and colour, skin tone. Less obviously, we inherit things like blood type or some diseases, like cystic fibrosis. In addition, severe trauma that our parents or grandparents experience can be stored in their bodies so that when they have children, part of that trauma is passed down. Research tells us that trauma is intergenerationally passed on through epigenetic mechanisms – parts of our DNA and genes.[9] It can seem surreal that trauma – something that affects our mental health – could be passed down physically. However, consider how much of the Defence Cascade is about our body's physical response to trauma. Sexual abuse, as with many traumas, happens to our bodies; it makes sense then, that it can be passed down from parent to child.

The behaviour we inherit through intergenerational trauma can be more tangible. Traumatic events experienced by one generation (such as forced immigration, war, or abuse) can be passed down to its descendants through various means, such as changes in behaviour, parenting styles, and disproportionate emotional responses. The trauma experienced by parents or grandparents can impact the mental and emotional health of their children and grandchildren, even if these younger generations did not directly experience the traumatic events themselves. For an example, see below.

First generation (grandparent)

The grandparent experiences severe trauma, such as war, extreme poverty, or forced immigration. As a result, they become overly protective and anxious, constantly worrying about the safety of their family but unable to enjoy parenting or emotionally express love and affection for their children as they grow.

Second generation (parent)

Growing up with an overly protective but emotionally unavailable parent, the second generation develops a strict and controlling parenting style. They closely monitor their children's activities to prevent any harm, mirroring the vigilance they experienced with their own parent. They might also develop certain health behaviours, like alcoholism, to help cope with the emotional deficits they experienced from their parent and, on an unconscious level, the emotional connection they may still desire with them.

Third generation (child)

The third-generation child, raised in a highly controlled environment, inherits a heightened sense of anxiety. They might constantly feel uneasy or hypervigilant and, at the same time, look for parental figures outside of the family due to their parent's alcoholism. This might make them vulnerable to people who would take advantage of their need for parent figures. The child goes through life on the lookout for danger and desiring someone to protect them, unaware of the impact of the grandparent's trauma on them.

Much like individual trauma, different circumstances can exacerbate intergenerational trauma for families, such as discrimination or a lack of financial resources, education, or job opportunities. In fact, whole communities can be affected by intergenerational trauma. For example, working-class areas impacted by generational poverty and diasporic groups (any group of people that has been dispersed outside its traditional homeland, either involuntarily or by migration) can face disproportionate amounts of trauma that echo through generations.

I want to acknowledge that facing intergenerational trauma does not mean you are destined to pass it on to younger generations. Trauma in your heritage does *not* predetermine your relationships or parenting skills. It can, however, present challenges that others may not fully understand and that require your energy to manage.

I work with many men who have experienced intergenerational trauma. In the chaos of traumatised families, sexual abuse often goes unnoticed. It becomes the survivor's job to not just work on their own recovery, but also to unravel the trauma of abuse, poverty, war, slavery, or asylum-seeking from generations gone by.

2.3   Men, trauma and sexual abuse: Where are we now?

When looking for facts, support services, research papers, or even literature, film, or other media on sexual abuse, the subject of abuse towards females is far more prevalent than anything addressing male survivors. This is not surprising, as the number of female sexual assault survivors outweighs that of male survivors. There has been pushback to the lack of male representation in the area of survivors of sexual violence. Some men's rights activists have framed this gender divide as a simplistic 'us vs them' scenario and accuse feminists of erasing the victimisation of men, via moral panic over the feminist concept of rape culture.[10] Within this book, there is no such comparison. It is precisely because of feminist scholars, community leaders, survivors, and therapists that therapeutic interventions for all genders are starting to improve, albeit slowly.

In addition to (or because of) this work by feminists, society has taken a bigger interest in stories of abuse against males. This includes fictional accounts like the UK soap opera *Hollyoaks*, which first tackled the subject of male rape in 2000 and then again in 2014. The UK's longest running soap opera, *Coronation Street*, dealt with male rape in 2018, generating 200 complaints to Ofcom, the UK's communications regulator.[11] In 2020, the television limited series *I May Destroy You* premiered on the BBC and HBO. Set in London, it featured a mainly Black British cast and examined female and male rape as well as 'stealthing', the act of removing a condom during sex without the other person's consent, considered rape according to English and Welsh law. In 2022, the soap *Eastenders* consulted with male sexual abuse charities to run a male rape story. The year I'm writing, 2024, saw the release of *Baby Reindeer*, a show created by comedian Richard Gadd about abuse he suffered from a female stalker and a male perpetrator. The show's success saw huge spikes in first-time callers looking for support from UK male sexual abuse charities.

Recent high-profile news stories have also raised awareness. The conviction of Reynhard Sinaga between 2019 and 2020 for the rapes of 44 men (though it is suspected the real number of victims is in the 200s) in Manchester, UK, brought the topic into mainstream discussion. A number of abusive public figures in the US and UK have made headlines. In 2022, for example, the UK football sexual abuse scandal broke, with several former professional players speaking up about abuse they endured from coaches and sports scouts during the 1970s, 1980s, and 1990s. This involved 849 alleged victims, with 2,807 incidents spanning 340 different football clubs.

Despite the increased awareness, men still struggle to come forward and report sexual abuse. The reasons for this are multifaceted. For older gay men, the shadow of Section 28, a series of laws across Britain that banned the promotion of homo-sexuality by local authorities, is still felt when talking about sexuality. Section 28 was introduced by Margaret Thatcher's Conservative government and lasted from 1988 to 2000 in Scotland and until 2003 in England and Wales. According to an entry of the Stonewall blog from November 2003, Section 28

> had deprived generations of LGBT pupils the chance of seeing people like them in the books, plays, leaflets or films their schools could stock or show. Teachers weren't allowed to teach about same-sex relationships; anyone who broke the law could face disciplinary action.[12]

The generation of gay men affected by Section 28 is also the generation robbed of gay elders due to the AIDS epidemic. Many of the gay male survivors I see for therapy remember the legacy of this law and the stigma towards gay sex as 'dirty', which still prevents them from feeling open to having conversations about sexual abuse they have suffered. Ideas about masculinity that include stigma towards male survivors are common in society, including the criminal justice system. In fact, all survivors of historic sexual abuse, regardless of gender, can find society dis-misses it or fails to take it seriously. In 2019, British writer and politician Boris Johnson described the money police spent on non-recent child abuse investigations as 'spaffed up a wall'.[13] Months after making this statement, he was elected as British Prime Minister.

Relationships between the police and marginalised groups such as Black and gay communities have always been difficult. In 2023, Baroness Louise Casey was com-missioned to review the Metropolitan Police (Met), Britain's largest police force, in the wake of the Sarah Everard kidnap, rape, and murder by an off-duty police officer. Casey's review found that the Met police were institutionally racist, misogynist, and homophobic.[14] These are hardly the conditions under which most men would be will-ing to report sexual abuse. There are many examples of rape cases being mishandled or neglected even when the male victim does not belong to a minority group. It can be hard to find data on trans and nonbinary people's experiences of sexual abuse, but a 2015 survey of 27,715 trans respondents, conducted in the United States, tells us that nearly half of respondents (47 per cent) had been sexually assaulted at some point in their lifetime, and one in ten had been sexually assaulted that year. In Black trans communities, the numbers were higher: 53 per cent said they had been sexually assaulted in their lifetime and 13 per cent in the last year.[15]

Other groups it can be hard to find information on include men who experience honour-based abuse, in which men can be forced into marriage and sexual relation-ships for a number of reasons, including strengthening family ties, securing visas, or attempting to 'cure' or hide gay or trans identities. Men with learning difficulties are also targeted for honour-based abuse. Data from the joint Home Office and Foreign and Commonwealth Office Forced Marriage Unit shows that in cases in 2017 that involved a victim with learning difficulties, just over half (55 per cent) were male.

Reading all this as a male survivor of sexual abuse, it may be hard not to feel bleak. If you are an ally who supports a male survivor, it may be hard not to feel overwhelmed. However, more survivors are speaking out, and slowly but surely, different parts of society are listening. Be it in the criminal justice system or TV shows, a greater sense is emerging that change needs to come if we are to provide care for male survivors and keep men and boys safe in the future. I genuinely believe that you are part of that change too. As survivors, we are used to 'getting on with it' and burying our emotions, but you have chosen to do something different. You have decided to shine a light on what may be some of the most painful and stigmatised parts of your life. You have started the process of working out what trauma means to you. If you are an ally, you have made a conscious choice to learn more about the person or people you support, rather than relying on myths and stigma to inform your opinions.

As we have seen, trauma looks different for everyone and there is no 'one-size-fits-all' to the recovery of trauma (if there were, it wouldn't be such a buzzword with thousands of self-help books on the topic). Gradually, it feels like we are approaching a tipping point where men, regardless of identity, will be able to find support for their trauma or sexual abuse experiences. By deciding you want something to change, you are part of that shift, and I think it's amazing.

Square Breathing

When to try this: Try this when you want to calm yourself down or need a moment of stillness

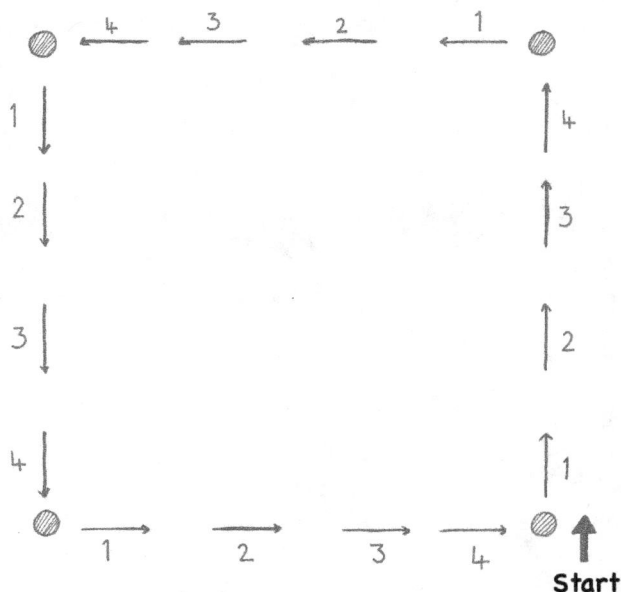

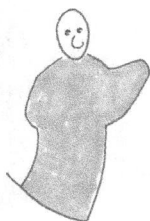

- Begin at the 'Start'. Breathe in (I breathe in and out through the nose, but do whatever is most comfortable for you). As you breathe in, follow the arrows upward counting up to 4.

- Once you get to the top, breathe out for 4, following the arrows from right to left.

- Now breathe in for 4, following the arrows downward.

- And finally, breathe out for 4, following the arrows back to the start. Repeat this as many times as you like.

This is Square Breathing. Practise doing this in your minds eye so you can do it anytime you need to feel calm or want to slow down your breathing

For A4 and printable versions of this worksheet, visit www.jeremysachs.com

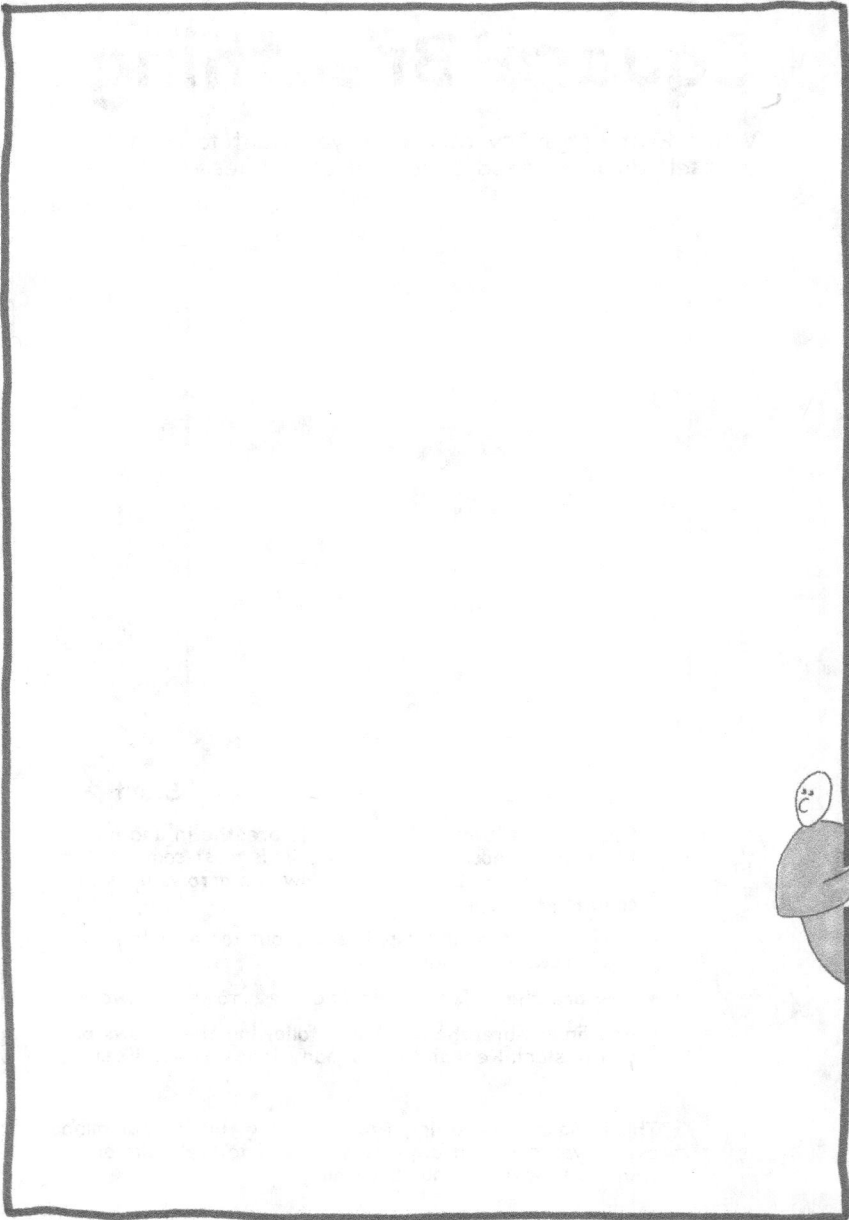

For A4 and printable versions of this worksheet, visit www.jeremysachs.com

Resources

Close to Home *by Michael Magee*

ISBN: 9780241582978
This novel, set in Belfast, explores themes of intergenerational trauma, poverty and sexual abuse. Despite the heavy subject matter, it is written in an accessible style that is not overly triggering. If you are looking for a book that delves into trauma without being too intense, this may be a good place to start.

The Trauma Talks by Jeremy Sachs and Katherine Cox

The Trauma Talks is my podcast. It explores a different experience of trauma each episode via people with lived experience, including men's experience of sexual abuse both in childhood and in adulthood. Search 'The Trauma Talks' wherever you listen to your podcasts.

Signposting

The Survivors Trust

https://thesurvivorstrust.org
An umbrella organisation supporting specialist rape and sexual abuse services in the voluntary sector.

1in6

https://1in6.org
Offers support and resources specifically for male survivors of sexual abuse and assault, including online support groups, a 24/7 helpline, and educational materials.

Notes

1 Nick Haslam, Brodie C. Dakin, Fabian Fabiano, Melanie J. McGrath, Joshua Rhee, Ekaterina Vylomova, et al., 'Harm inflation: Making sense of concept creep', *European Review of Social Psychology* 31, no. 1 (2020): 254–286, doi:10.1080/10463283.2020.1796080.
2 Gabor Maté, 'The trauma doctor: Gabor Maté on happiness, hope, and how to heal our deepest wounds', *The Guardian*, 12 April 2023. www.theguardian.com/lifeandstyle/2023/apr/12/the-trauma-doctor-gabor-mate-on-happiness-hope-and-how-to-heal-our-deepest-wounds, accessed 28 May 2024.
3 'Numbing the pain: Survivors' voices of childhood sexual abuse and addiction', One in Four, 2019. oneinfour.org.uk/wp-content/uploads/2019/03/RackMultipart20190320-8959-khxw2x.pdf, accessed 2 August 2024.
4 Kasia Kozlowska, Peter Walker, Loyola McLean, and Pascal Carrive, 'Fear and the defense cascade: Clinical implications and management', *Harvard Review of Psychiatry* 23, no. 4 (2015): 263–287.

5 Joseph E. LeDoux, 'The neurocircuitry of fear, anxiety, and stress: Implications for mental health', *Neuron* 37, no. 1 (2003): 12–25, doi:10.1016/S0896-6273(02)01143-4.
6 Muriel A. Hagenaars, John F. Stins and Karin Roelofs, 'Aversive life events enhance human freezing responses', *Journal of Experimental Psychology: General*, no. 141 (2012): 98–105.
7 H. Stefan Bracha, 'Freeze, flight, fight, fright, faint: Adaptationist perspectives on the acute stress response spectrum', *CNS Spectrums* 9 (2004): 679–685.
8 Thema Bryant-Davis, 'The Cultural context of trauma recovery: Considering the post-traumatic stress disorder practice guideline and intersectionality', *Psychotherapy (Chic)* 56, no. 3 (2019): 400–408, doi:10.1037/pst0000241.
9 Shui Jiang, Lynne Postovit, Annamaria Cattaneo, ElisabethB. Binder, and Katherine J. Aitchison, 'Epigenetic modifications in stress response genes associated with childhood trauma', *Frontiers in Psychiatry* 10 (2019): doi: 10.3389/fpsyt.2019.00808.
10 Lise Gotell and Emily Dutton 'Sexual violence in the "manosphere": Antifeminist men's rights discourses on rape', *International Journal for Crime, Justice and Social Democracy* 5, no. 2 (2016): 65–80, https://doi.org/10.5204/ijcjsd.v5i2.310.
11 David Brown, 'Ofcom rules on Coronation Street David Platt rape storyline after 200 complaints', *Radio Times*, 8 May 2018. www.radiotimes.com/tv/soaps/coronation-str eet/ofcom-rules-on-coronation-street-david-platt-rape-storyline-after-200-complaints, accessed 2 August 2024.
12 '18 November 2003: Section 28 bites the dust', Stonewall, 2024. www.stonewall.org. uk/our-work/campaigns/18-november-2003-section-28-bites-dust, accessed 2 August 2024.
13 Dan Sabbagh, 'Boris Johnson under fire over remarks about child abuse inquiries', *The Guardian*, 13 March 2019. www.theguardian.com/politics/2019/mar/13/boris-johnson-under-fire-over-remarks-about-child-abuse-inquiries, accessed 2 August 2024.
14 Baroness Casey of Blackstock DBE CB, *Baroness Casey Review: Final Report: An Independent Review into the Standards of Behaviour and Internal Culture of the Metropolitan Police Service* (London: Metropolitan Police, March 2023). www.met.pol ice.uk/SysSiteAssets/media/downloads/met/about-us/baroness-casey-review/update-march-2023/baroness-casey-review-march-2023a.pdf, accessed 2 August 2024.
15 Sandy E. James, Jody L. Herman, Susan Rankin, Mara Keisling, Lisa Mottet, and Ma'ayan Anafi, *The Report of the 2015 U.S. Transgender Survey* (Washington, DC: National Center for Transgender, 2016). https://transequality.org/sites/default/files/docs/usts/USTS%20Full%20Report%20-%20FINAL%201.6.17.pdf, accessed 2 August 2024.

Chapter 3

Trauma vs everyday life

Chapter Contents

My trauma

The trauma affects every part of my life. Sometimes it feels like it's written on my forehead in Sharpie so everyone can see it. I struggle with intense anxiety and depression. There are days when I don't want to get out of bed. I have cycles of flashbacks and nightmares and certain sights, sounds, or even smells can trigger vivid memories of the abuse. I also get aches and pains and fatigue. Doctors say it's due to stress, but I think it's the trauma, too.

I often feel overwhelming emotions like shame, even though I know, logically, it wasn't my fault. These feelings are compounded by being a Black gay man. There are cultural expectations that come with my identity, and hardly anyone who looks like me has had similar experiences. My relationships suffer, and intimacy is particularly challenging; physical closeness can trigger panic attacks or dissociation. I fear that any partner I might have won't fully understand or might become frustrated with my reactions, or they might blame themselves, and that would feel even worse for me.

I've had to find the money for private therapy because the therapy I had on the NHS was brief, and while it was helpful in some ways, it didn't feel like they were going to 'get it' – this might be unfair on the therapist, but it's definitely how I felt. Private therapy is expensive, and I'm lucky my job pays well; I couldn't have afforded it a few years ago. I also do stretches in the morning and try to stay active – this helps the physical symptoms of trauma.

DOI: 10.4324/9781003423331-3

> Each day, I work towards embracing my identity and finding strength in my resilience. Despite the ongoing challenges, I am committed to healing and to helping others who might be facing similar struggles.
>
> Anonymous survivor

3.1   Brains, behaviour, and life after abuse

Our brains are mysterious, wonderful things. They can surprise us day or night. Smells can invoke fond memories, dreams can stir up powerful emotions, and songs can conjure feelings from the past. All of this while it automatically keeps us breathing, our heart pumping, and our body moving. Michio Kaku, a theoretical physicist, said, 'The human brain has 100 billion neurons, each neuron connected to 10,000 other neurons. Sitting on your shoulders is the most complicated object in the known universe'. A wonderful (and daunting) quote. Brains also have the remarkable ability to adapt to all sorts of environments. In fact, the brain starts adapting from the very earliest moments in our lives.

While we are babies growing in the womb, our organs and bodily systems are developing, preparing for life outside the womb when we are born. At the point of birth, our lungs breathe air, our nervous system senses sensations, our kidneys clean our blood, and our digestive system draws energy from milk. However, one organ that is relatively underdeveloped at birth is the brain. This is because one of the brain's jobs is to adapt to the environment we are born into. A baby's senses – touch, smell, sight, hearing, taste – all gather information about the outside world and feed that information to the brain. Then the brain decides how to adapt to the outside world based on that information. This is part of a phenomenon called *neuroplasticity* – the process of the brain reorganising as we grow. If a baby is born into a family that meets their needs and keeps them safe and loved, then the brain adapts to a safe environment. However, a baby or a child growing up in an unsafe environment where there is sustained threat, violence, or need will often have to adapt to that. These infants and children, despite being in survival mode almost constantly, are rarely able to identify the danger they are in. This is because the unsafe environment is all they know; why would they expect any different? In addition, they are hard-wired to love their parents or caregivers. It is almost impossible for a child to think a parent isn't deserving of their love. It is only looking back as teenagers or adults that they realise they were vulnerable and needed to adapt to dangerous people or difficult environments. Many survivors of sexual abuse remember experiencing the world in a way that is different to their peers. Someone who grew up in a household where they were unsafe might report

- Having a heightened awareness of where people are in the home
- Being able to intuitively read the moods and emotions of people around them

- Having a heightened alertness to threat
- Being able to make themselves almost 'invisible' while moving through their home to avoid attention (a common example of this is children who know which floorboard or stair is squeaky and avoid stepping on it to so as not draw attention to themselves)
- Having a sensitivity, as older children or adults, to whether other people have experienced similar trauma
- Developing a rich inner world where they retreat, rather than seeking comfort in a parent or friend
- Having a nervousness towards other adults, even if they are caring (like a teacher); alternatively, some report seeking out other adults to form close relationships with

Living in constant survival mode takes its toll on the body and brain. The body releases stress hormones in response to danger, but if this keeps happening, the stress hormones can stick around in our bodies even after the danger has passed. This means that children, teenagers, and adults who have experienced sexual abuse can continue to have traumatic responses throughout their lives in everyday situations. Survivors can find themselves stuck in survival mode. Being stuck like this in everyday life can have an enormous impact on survivors' lives. They may struggle in education more than their peers or find themselves having disproportionally emotional reactions at work. Personal relationships may be full of conflict, arguments, and emotional pain, or the idea of any type of relationship may be so anxiety-inducing that survivors avoid them altogether. On top of this, many survivors from minority communities experience a phenomenon called *minority stress*.[1] This occurs when minoritised people facing discrimination, stigma, and prejudice feel additional societal stress from the added challenges of being a member of a minority group, along with internalised stigma, homophobia, or shame. Societal discrimination, self-stigma, and sexual trauma can be a complex combination and cause great stress to a person's mental and physical state.

To figure out whether - parts of us are stuck in survival mode, it can help to look at ways we experience ourselves in the world. Below is a list of nine ways survivors may respond to their trauma on a daily basis.

1. Window of tolerance

A person *without* a history of trauma may tolerate everyday stressors like late trains, exam pressure, job interviews, and relationship strain well. They have a good-sized window of tolerance, meaning their tolerance for stress is high. They can go about everyday activities feeling like *I've got this!* and everything is manageable. This is called the *optimal arousal zone*. For survivors, this may be more difficult. Due to the impact of sexual abuse, we may have a smaller window of tolerance and find everyday stresses disproportionally difficult. A small stress will feel bigger to us, and a big stress can feel unmanageable.

Stress can push those with a smaller window of tolerance out of their window in two different directions. Some survivors will be pushed into hyper-arousal, whereas others will be pushed into hypo-arousal.

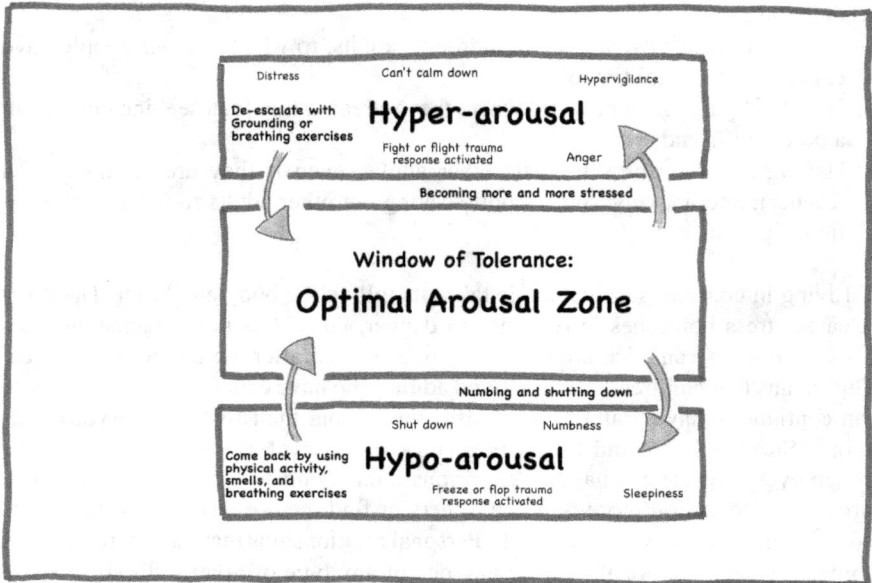

Below shows the difference between the responses.

Hyper-arousal

- Fight or flight trauma response activated
- Impaired or rigid thinking, often accompanied by racing thoughts
- Lots of emotions or emotional reactions to situations
- Distress, hypervigilance, panic, or anger

Hypo-arousal

- Freeze or flop trauma response activated
- Feelings start to shut off or become emotionally numb
- Absence of sensations
- Becomes isolated or withdraws
- Depression, hopelessness, sleepiness, or emptiness

Interestingly, and disturbingly for those who experience it, both hyper- and hypo-arousal can lead to dissociation (see number 8 in this list). Those who become hyper-aroused require soothing and gentle grounding in the present moment.

Those who become hypo-aroused need gentle stimulation to bring them back to the here-and-now.

I often encourage those working with survivors to agree on a smell they can use to ground survivors if they dissociate. This could be an essential oil, hand cream, etc. Often, smells cut through dissociation and can reorient a person. (It's important to decide what smell to use beforehand, as some smells may have strong negative associations).

2. Hypervigilance

A brain that has adapted to sustained abuse, violence, or threat can become hyper-vigilant over time. This occurs when we go about our day in a state of increased alertness and sensitivity to our surroundings. It's common for people who experienced a difficult childhood to feel hypervigilant. Survivors' brains learn to be sensitive to danger, which initially occurs as a survival strategy while in abusive or dangerous situations and can become habitual after danger passes, constantly sensing danger in everyday environments, even when there is none. Along with feeling hypervigilant, some survivors have fantasies that justify the feeling of danger. Some imagine people they know acting towards them in violent ways – a flatmate bursts into the room to attack them, a friend is aggressively violent – even when, logically, they know this would never happen. Others imagine being the victim of violence at the hands of strangers as they go about their everyday lives.

Many people from marginalised groups will also be familiar with hypervigilance. A person can become hypervigilant when they experience discrimination, learn to expect rejection and prejudice-related events like hate crimes, and have to conceal aspects of their identity. This is part of the experience of minority stress, which can often compound trauma. It can be difficult for both the survivor and the therapist to unpack the effects of hypervigilance in the therapy room, as a lifetime of varying threats and violence can become enmeshed in everyday experiences.

3. Memory

Trauma can affect how we store or access our memories, particularly of traumatic events, though for each survivor this can differ drastically. We can be left with patchy memories, full graphic scenes in our mind's eye, or we can forget instances altogether. Some will look back on their lives and only traumatic memories will stand out. These memories are bright and loud and difficult and can cause everyday or happy memories to fade away or feel emotionally distant. This is common with those of us who survive childhood abuse, even if we were looked after and loved sometimes: the abusive memories are more accessible.

Memory and language

Memories, particularly early ones, are a product of collective experience. As children, we don't necessarily hold independent memories of what has happened to us. Families collectively reinforce memories. They use language to refer to and strengthen childhood experiences. For example, a father may say to his child, 'Remember when we went to the seaside? You played with your red bucket and a seagull stole your brother's ice cream?'

The child in this scenario could have been too young to remember this or even understand what the event means; an infant is unlikely to remember a seagull if they are too young to know what a seagull is. However, because the family reinforce this memory by talking about it through the years, it becomes held collectively. The parents revisit this memory every summer before the annual trip to the beach. They laugh about it and might even look at photographs. Through this process, the children understand the memories and emotions discussed: the love for the red bucket, the peril of a bold seagull stealing ice cream. The memory lives in the collective memory of the family, rather than independently with the child.

When sexual abuse happens in early life, the memories are not generally reinforced in this way. The abuse is often secret and unspoken. Over a lifetime, these painful memories can become foggy and distant or even seem to disappear. The survivor's memories have not been reinforced, and they may therefore lose the memory. Often, however, they hold on to a deep sense of disturbance that can manifest in many ways in later life, such as depression, anxiety, or shame, as well as difficulty maintaining relationships or jobs.

Memories may also fade or be hard to access in cases where abuse happens at a very young age, when the survivor may not understand or have language for what is happening to them. They might feel the abuse is unwanted without conceptually understanding the experience. This abuse at a pre-verbal age can remain buried for decades.

For those of us abused in adulthood or adolescence, memories can also be difficult to access. When we have a trauma response, the parts of our brain responsible for processing and storing new memories switches off. Imagine a fire alarm going off in a building. Suddenly everyone stops what they are doing, puts down their daily tasks, and heads for safety. The same thing happens in our brain. A traumatic event activates the internal fire alarm, and our brain stops its daily task (of processing and memorising events) in order to prioritise survival. This means when we look back at a traumatic event, trying to piece together what happened, it can be difficult to remember. Both the traumatic event and the hours before and after can seem foggy.

4. Flashbacks

Flashbacks can be part of our dreaming or sleep state, but we can also experience them when we are awake. They can be a sudden memory intruding into our consciousness or a feeling of dread, like an emotional memory, rather than one we can picture. Other flashbacks can be experienced in our body rather than our mind, as when we suddenly experience a touch, smell or taste that brings us back to a distressing state.

5. Sleep

Sleep is essential to our wellbeing, yet it is often one of the first things to be disrupted when life gets tricky or trauma comes to the surface. As survivors, our relationship with sleep can be complicated. On top of that, very little is known about sleep generally or how to improve it. We hear a lot about good sleep hygiene techniques, but when they don't work, it can leave survivors with nowhere to go. A lack of sleep doesn't just mean we are exhausted in the daytime. It can affect our cognitive functioning – how we think and process information – and it means our immune system doesn't get the chance to rest and recover from the day, leading us to feel run-down or ill. Some people might have the opposite issue, sleeping for eight or nine hours a night and still finding it difficult to feel awake. They may want to stay in bed and struggle to get up.

Common sleep issues survivors can face include

- **Too little sleep.** This can be categorised as insomnia, disrupted or fractured sleep, inability to fall asleep, or constantly waking up at night.
- **Too much sleep.** This can include an inability to get up in the morning, going to bed in the day if things get difficult or using sleep to avoid difficult feelings or to kill time.
- **Waking in the mornings with a feeling of dread.** This can be defined as a sense of dread and overwhelm about the day from the moment you wake up or extreme fantasies about getting into accidents or experiencing bereavements to avoid the day ahead; either way, the day feels like too much and staying in bed can feel like the only option.
- **Nightmares.** Nightmares may or may not be specifically about the abuse, but are troubling and frightening and may feel like past traumas or abuse; some may be old memories rising up from survivors' subconscious or position survivors as an abuser or having sexual encounters that they would not want in real life; survivors may wake in the night or early morning feeling terrible or terrified by intrusive thoughts or memories flooding in.
- **Broken sleep.** For some survivors, sleep can be broken in the night; they may wake either because their body simply can't remain asleep or because they are disturbed by multiple nightmares, and this can happen many times over the course of a night.

6. Depression, anxiety, or both

If you're reading this book as an ally or survivor, it will come as no surprise to you that depression and anxiety are common among survivors of abuse. While depression and anxiety are also high among the general population, a study conducted in China found that young male survivors of childhood abuse were not only either depressed or anxious, but they also experienced guilt and suicidal ideation.[2]

It is normal for survivors to have feelings of sadness or hopelessness, regardless of whether the sexual abuse was a long time ago or recent. It's also normal to feel anxious after abuse, sense that things might go wrong, exist in a constant state of 'what if...' or disproportionally worry about outcomes. Male survivors are used to simply 'getting on with it', particularly if we experience depression or anxiety over long periods of time. It may not even occur to us that these feelings are linked to abuse; we just accept them as a fact of life.

Depression and anxiety are treatable, either with therapy, medication, or a mix of both. Some survivors may feel that if they go to a doctor for help with these, they will need to disclose the sexual abuse, and this stops them seeking help. The truth is, you do not need to disclose abuse, even to a GP, if you don't want to. It is normal for people to seek help managing depression and anxiety. Of course, if you are thinking about disclosing abuse to your GP, that's okay too. If you are thinking about disclosing to a healthcare professional but don't know where to start, take a look at Chapter 9 on disclosure.

7. Anger

Male survivors often hear that they have 'anger issues' or need to 'get anger management training'. They can be told this by friends, loved ones, or colleagues. Whether or not the advice is well intentioned, it rarely helps the survivor. In fact, it can make things worse or lead to feelings of shame, and this becomes a trap, leaving survivors saying, 'I feel shamed, so get angry, and get angry, so feel shamed'.

In most cases, the anger a survivor feels is an entirely appropriate reaction; however, the anger the survivor feels might not be appropriate given the circumstances. For a lot of us, this makes sense. During abuse or rape, we are unlikely to feel anger, let alone get the chance to express it. Our brain and body are too busy surviving for us to be angry. However, as the days, months, and years go by, we start to feel anger about the abuse. We can feel angry at the people around us who should have protected us. We can feel angry towards society when it doesn't take us seriously, towards the person/s who abused us, and (sometimes most easily) at ourselves for allowing it to happen. While the anger can feel uncontrollable, we are in a safer environment compared to the trauma state when we were abused; therefore, the anger is safe enough to come out. Despite that, it may still feel so painful or shameful to be angry directly at the abuse that the anger comes out at different things. We can feel angry at the people who love us, ourselves, strangers on the train, or people in power. In fact, we may get angry at the whole world to avoid the pain of being angry at the sexual abuse. It is easy to see how survivors with a small window of tolerance might experience anger, then shame, then anger again at the shame, in a constant cycle. Some of us experience our anger 'explosively' – we are more prone to road rage, arguments, throwing objects across the room – and others of us experience our anger 'implosively' – we are more prone to passive-aggressive responses or store our anger up until later. Others of us can ruminate for days on anger-inducing experiences.

For still others, anger feels inaccessible. We don't get angry – or rather, we cannot access our anger. We forgive people or say we are not bothered by wrongs that should be anger-inducing. This can confuse the people around us, leaving loved ones asking, 'Why aren't you annoyed?' at some wrongdoing. I have met survivors who told me that expressing anger as a child meant inviting severe punishment, meaning that they never developed the ability to be appropriately angry, so their anger lies dormant. Others say that to be angry puts them in touch with such deep pain that it becomes too uncontrollable and they become rageful. This type of inaccessible anger can make us feel like we are stuck; our emotions collapse in on themselves, leaving us numb, stuck, or depressed. People who report this may also feel stuck in parts of their lives: at work, in relationships or even in therapy.

We can forget that anger is a natural human emotion. It is an appropriate response in the face of injustice, violation of boundaries, or when someone harms us or someone we love. As a survivor, you have every right to be angry about what happened to you.

8. Dissociation

Dissociation can happen when a person feels overwhelmed. We can experience it in different ways, including losing time or having gaps in memory, numbness or detachment from our emotions, or a sense that we are acting like a different person some of the time. This can be brought on by a traumatic memory, everyday stresses such as exam pressure, work deadlines, an argument, or anything that threatens to emotionally overwhelm us.

Some experience dissociation as a comforting place to go to in their minds. When they face emotional challenges, they start to shut down and go somewhere foggy, quiet, and away from the stress. Other people describe dissociation as a terrifying place. I have seen people I've worked with for over five years dissociate and not recognise me. Some may feel that coming *out* of a state of dissociation may risk death. I've sat with clients on the floor, hearing them tell me that if they leave their dissociated state, they feel like they will be destroyed.

Some dissociation can happen even without our knowing. It can feel like getting sleepy, staring into space or zoning out. The different experiences and severities of dissociation are huge.

9. Triggers

It is common to hear the term *being triggered*. A lot of psychological language is finding its way into everyday use. Generally, I think this is a good thing. It helps people describe their experiences and gets conversations going about mental health that would not have happened in the past. The downside to this, however, is that the phrase has also been used to mock or bully people in public forums. In a psychological setting, the term refers to an event that causes a trauma response, which can be severely distressing for the person triggered. It can result in anger, fear, panic, or complete shutdown or dissociation. It doesn't have to be a new life-threatening situation. In fact, it can be anything from a smell, song, or colour to the way people treat us; because a lot of survivors are hypervigilant, we can be sensitive to threats, even if they are not real, and this can trigger a trauma response. You'll find that in this book, I use the word *activated* more than *triggered*. I do this to avoid any of the nasty associations that have developed through bullying misuse of the word *triggered*. Plus, I think *activated* is actually very descriptive. When activated – or triggered – our brain is literally activating survival mode, getting ready to use fight, flight, or whatever is needed to survive.

Any one of these trauma symptoms can be disturbing. However, it is likely that sexual abuse survivors experience more than one. This can be isolating. We can feel like we are 'crazy' and the only ones who experience the world in this way. It is important for us to know that these symptoms are normal reactions to the *abnormal* situations we have survived. Because our brain and body were under such severe threat, they used powerful methods of surviving – so powerful, in fact, that they linger in our body, just in case we are threatened again. This means the everyday world can be harder for us to manage than it is for people who have not needed such extreme survival tactics. I really want you to know that you are not alone in feeling and reacting as you do.

3.2   Finding your words

Those of us who have sought help from mental health professionals can find clinical or medical language useful. It can add weight to our disturbing experiences and provide a framework of language to describe them. However, this approach is not for everyone. For some of us, clinical or medical language can feel oppressive or sterile or fail to accurately sum up how we feel. Others may have never found an opportunity to put into words how they feel about their abuse, and using clinical language might feel too overwhelming.

For men, finding language that can appropriately summarise our everyday experiences of living with trauma can be powerful. Not only does it help us to conceptualise how we are thinking and feeling, but it also gives us the power to communicate this to other people. For some survivors, this is a huge step. If clinical or medical language feels like it's not for you, or if you are at the beginning of your recovery, it can help to think of creative ways of communicating your experience. You may start this by considering metaphors or similes. Metaphors and similes are not literal but symbolic, using comparison to express abstract ideas so that most people will understand without needing too much explanation. A metaphor compares two things by saying that one thing *is* (figuratively) another thing, whereas a simile says one thing *is like* another thing.

Metaphors, for example, include

- My sadness is a dark hole in my chest that is black and deep.
- The shame is dissolving my stomach.
- Feeling the grass between my toes is my religious experience.

Examples of similes include

- Feeling understood is like feeling the warm sun on your face.
- When I have to speak to strangers I feel like a child.
- When I wake up from a bad dream it's like a thunderstorm in my brain.

It doesn't matter whether you use metaphors or similes. What matters is that you find ways of communicating that feel right for you.

There are some common metaphors and similes that I hear survivors use regularly to explain what it is like to live with the aftermath of sexual abuse. You may already use some of these. If so, it can be useful to see you're not alone in using them; many people have sat in front of me and used these to describe the indescribable. It is also possible that this is the first time you have seen these and they capture your experience.

Wearing a mask

Many survivors identify with wearing a mask. They can sustain relationships, go out with friends, hold jobs, and do all the things they need to do in life. However, for survivors this can take energy. They can put on a mask for the world to see, but underneath they feel isolated, numb, or full of anxiety.

Wearing a mask constantly is exhausting. It can create a disconnect with survivors' authentic selves. They can spend so much time either masking their traumatic symptoms or having to act in certain ways due to prejudice that it can become difficult to nurture a true self or find spaces where they can relax and be themselves. Similarly, autistic people can find themselves 'masking', while members of minority communities often 'code switch'. These are complex types of masks that can be part of a survival mechanism that intersects with the stress of sexual abuse.

Masking

Masking, for autistic and other neurodivergent people, involves consciously or unconsciously suppressing or altering natural behaviours and responses to fit into societal expectations. This can include mimicking neurotypical social cues, hiding stimming behaviours (repetitive movements or sounds), forcing eye contact, and suppressing personal interests or preferences to avoid standing out. While masking can help neurodivergent individuals navigate social situations, it can also lead to significant stress, exhaustion, and mental health issues over time. This becomes particularly problematic when neurodivergent people reach out for psychological support to manage trauma symptoms. They can be accused of behaving inappropriately or have their abuse experience questioned when not performing victimhood or showing emotions in a way neurotypical people think they should.

Code switching

Many people from minority backgrounds code switch. Similar to masking, code switching occurs when a person adjusts their language, syntax, and behaviour depending on their environment. It's similar to using 'a phone voice' that differs from your day-to-day speaking voice. The difference is that code switching is a conscious or unconscious action taken by a member of an underrepresented group. It's an attempt to fit into the dominant culture by becoming more acceptable to that culture. In the context of survivors, many men from minoritised groups feel the need to code switch in order to access healthcare, communicating their needs in ways that healthcare providers (often members of the dominant culture) will understand and find acceptable. It is often exhausting for people from minority backgrounds to do this, as failing to code switch can result in not getting the care they need and successfully code switching can feel like validating negative stereotypes. It can result in people feeling like their authentic selves are unacceptable and that they need to conform to the dominant culture.

The box

Some memories are so difficult that we have no choice but to try and forget about them. The brain locks memories out of our consciousness until something difficult triggers them back into our awareness. 'The box' is the place we store these memories. Boxes make a good metaphor because they have lids, locks and keys and come in all shapes and sizes.

Sometimes we can feel like our box's lid is not closed properly and painful memories keep spilling out. Life events can knock the box over and everything can fall out. Alternatively, we can choose to open the box when we feel ready. Everybody's box looks different. Some are plain wooden boxes, some are antique trunks, others are cold hard and metal.

Behind the door

Some people describe feeling as if there is a whole version of them locked away, not just painful memories like with the box. It may be the traumatised version of them that they need to keep locked away, maybe because they are so angry that they want the whole world to burn. Or they could be so sensitive they find meaning in anything, from a look on the street to a hug that lasts a little too long. Whatever it is, behind the door is a version of them that is not completely trustworthy in public.

Getting in contact with that version of yourself can be risky. Therefore, the door is useful. You can shout through a door, peek through the keyhole, open it on a security chain, or kick it down in a crisis.

Inner child/inner parent

The concept of the inner child is useful for survivors who have been harmed in childhood. I also find it useful because I believe we all have within us a version of ourselves from every age we have ever been. If we find ourselves disproportionately affected by something like an argument with a friend, it could be because our inner child has been wounded by this event. The adult part of us might want to move on from the argument, but the child in us cannot get over the wound inflicted. We might feel abandoned and frightened by the argument, reminiscent of childhood experiences of abandonment. We may continue to feel wounded for months or years; even if the adult version of us has decided to move on, we may still hold on to the pain of the argument. This might mean that our inner child hasn't been soothed.

Abuse in childhood can leave our inner child underdeveloped. They may feel robbed of the opportunity to learn how to play, be creative, or experience curiosity with the world. As adults, this might affect their sex life, how they behave around friends in social situations, or how they interact with children. Their inner child lacks the skills to communicate their needs or know that the world can be safe. For survivors, developing an inner parent can be useful, helping us learn to self-soothe and tell ourselves we are safe. This can be challenging, as many reading this book will have never experienced good enough parenting and, instead, will have internalised critical or harsh parenting. Instead of soothing our inner child, our inner parent chastises or ignores us. We internalise our own abusive or neglectful parent's voice and use it on ourselves, telling ourselves we are stupid or worthless.

As survivors, we often need to not only re-parent our inner child but also develop new, kinder skills for our inner parent. This requires that we work to make up for the childhood we missed out on and learn how to parent in a way our own parents couldn't teach us.

Turning up and down the volume

In my therapy room, I often talk about trauma as a volume. When a survivor first comes to therapy, a lot of their daily life is drowned out by the volume of trauma. I explain that therapy can't undo what has happened, but it can help to turn down the volume on trauma, hopefully giving the client more control over that volume, making space for new experiences and feelings.

Of course, different situations can affect the volume of past trauma. Something that activates a trauma symptom may turn the volume up to maximum. Over time, though, it's our goal to develop the skill to turn the volume down when we need to.

Stuck behind thick glass

Survivors often use the metaphor of being stuck behind thick glass because they can be surrounded by people but still feel isolated and alone. They can see life going on around them but feel removed from it in a way that is hard to describe. I always think of aquariums when I hear this. The glass you see in aquarium tanks gives the illusion you're right there next to the fish. In reality, this glass is incredibly thick to withstand the pressure of gallons of water. We are much more separated from the fish than we think we are. Trauma can do this to us, too. We may appear to be in the middle of crowded streets or elbow-to-elbow at the dinner table with friends, but in reality, we feel far away, holding on to immense pressure.

In a fog

The sense of being in a fog or having brain fog is common when people have experienced or are experiencing a lot of traumatic, activating, or stressful situations but still need to function every day. This could be considered a type of dissociation. When in a fog, many survivors know they are there. They can even talk about it with friends or their therapist. However, if you ask them how they feel or what emotions they are experiencing, they can't tell you. They stay in a fog, unable to see themselves or connect authentically with the world.

I also see people for whom the fog is a form of collapsed rage. They are unable to be angry with perpetrators or people who failed to protect them. When this sort of rage has nowhere to go, or when the rage is so big that it's too dangerous to allow out, it can collapse inward into the survivor and disappear in the fog.

Pressure cooker

Many survivors experience of lots of small stresses that build up inside them. It can be difficult to manage multiple everyday stresses, and they can build into one big reaction or explosion, like a pressure cooker. The way to stop a pressure cooker from exploding is to release a little bit of pressure every so often. In my groups, we dedicate a lot of time to finding ways of releasing pressure so we don't explode.

3.3   Adverse childhood experiences (ACEs) and the Drama Triangle

Hopefully the last chapter gave you some insight into what goes on in the body and mind while we are under traumatic stress, and this chapter has helped to illustrate some of the long-term impacts of surviving trauma.

It can also help to understand other bits of psychology or theory. Not only can this offer insight into our everyday challenges and how they link to the abuse, but it can also show us that we are not alone and many others experience similar struggles to ours. Below, I will introduce ACEs, an academic and social framework for understanding challenges (including sexual abuse) experienced in early life, and the Drama Triangle, a component of a type of psychology called transactional analysis (TA), which concerns how people interact with other people. I've found that survivors really value these theories, as they help survivors not only to make sense of their own relationships but also to understand those around them (for more on TA, see Chapter 6, page 114).

ACEs

ACEs are a relatively new way of thinking about trauma. They are often used in academic settings and social care. They are a way of quantifying the experiences a person had before the age of 18 that may lead to a challenging childhood or adolescence, as well as struggles and poor health outcomes in adulthood.

ACEs include all types of abuse as well as household dysfunctions, such as adults responsible for providing care (like parents, but also extended family or other important care figures), being a single parent/carer or divorced, growing up in poverty, being raised in care or having a parent living with addiction or mental illness. It is commonly thought that the more ACEs a person faces, the more potential difficulties they face, such as poor physical or mental health, risk-taking behaviours or complicated relationships with drugs or alcohol. ACEs are not always useful in therapy because they attempt to quantify a person's social and psychological struggles by using a series of life events. This can invite a hierarchy of 'who had it worse'. There can also be a danger of survivors feeling that ACEs predetermine poorer health outcomes, which can be unhelpful.

Still, ACEs can help us when thinking about the context in which the sexual abuse took place and each person's unique experience. They can show us how our environment may contribute, maintain, or add to the stress of trauma.

Examples of ACEs:

- Physical abuse
- Sexual abuse
- Emotional abuse
- Neglect
- Living with someone who abuses drugs
- Living with someone who abuses alcohol
- Exposure to domestic violence
- Living or having lived in poverty
- Experiencing food poverty
- Living or having lived in insecure housing

- Living with long-term health conditions or caring for someone who does
- Living with oppression towards yourself or your community, such as in the case of members of ethnic, gender or sexual minority groups or members of the disabled community
- Living with someone who has gone to prison or living with a family member in prison
- Living with someone with serious mental illness
- Losing a parent through divorce, death or abandonment

Many male survivors are good at minimising their experiences. We say to ourselves, *It wasn't that bad; we should get over it*, or tell ourselves that others 'had it worse'. Using ACEs, we can see our sexual abuse in the context in which it happened alongside other elements that made us vulnerable. ACEs show us that each person's trauma is unique. While there may be great similarities in abuse stories among male survivors, ACEs show that comparing our experiences is often unhelpful because our needs, challenges, and upbringing were all unique to us.

Even if you survived sexual abuse in adulthood, ACEs can be useful, because understanding our lives before the abuse can help us understand either why we were vulnerable to sexual abuse or why the aftermath is uniquely painful to us.

The Drama Triangle (Karpman Triangle)

The Drama Triangle,[3] sometimes called the Karpman Triangle, is a social model that aims to reflect how all humans can interact with one another, not just survivors. It was proposed by psychiatrist Stephen B. Karpman in 1968 and is part of the TA mode of psychology (see Chapter 6, page 114). Karpman used it to illustrate the ways in which complex interactions occur between people who are enmeshed in conflict or toxic relationships. People can be drawn into different roles in the triangle, feeding off of the energy the conflict creates and becoming trapped in a particular way of interacting with certain people. The three roles in the Drama Triangle are victim, rescuer, and persecutor. They are set in an inverse triangle, rescuer and persecutor on top and victim at the bottom point. It is important to remember that a person is not put in their role within the triangle by another person. Rather, they actively (but subconsciously) put themselves there through how they interact with another person. People can move around the triangle, inhabiting different states depending on their relationship with the people around them.

The Rescuer

Saves people they view as vulnerable. Works hard to offer help, even if this help is not asked for.

The Persecutor

Often unaware of their own power and how it affects those around them. Makes negative and often destructive comments about others, either intentionally or flippantly.

The Victim

Can be overwhelmed by their own vulnerability and struggles to take responsibility for their situation or help themselves. Often has a history of being victimised.

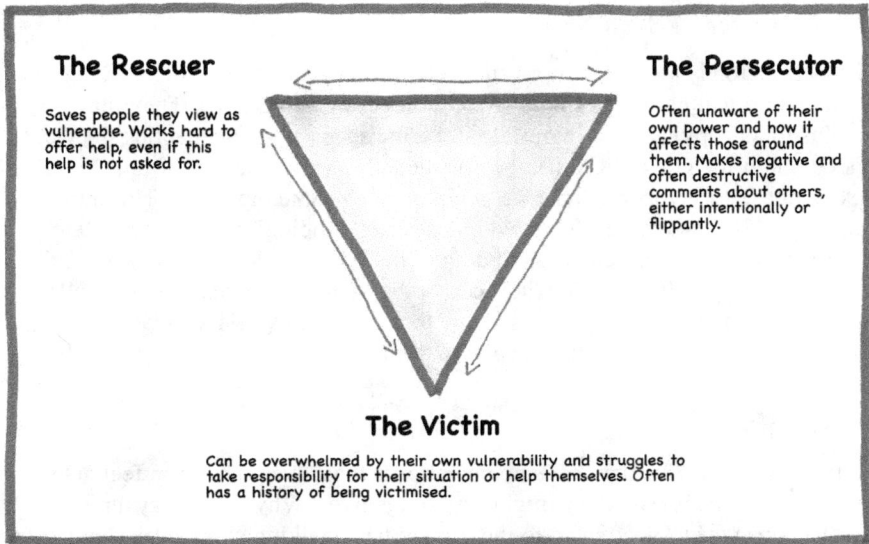

Here is a breakdown of the rescuer, persecutor and victim states.

The rescuer

The rescuer is a person who needs to help and support someone else, regardless of whether that help and support is needed or not. The rescuer may make caring a big part of their identity and get stuck in complicated relationships where they are the caregiver. This may be welcomed by the person receiving care, but it can also feel overbearing. A rescuer may feel guilty if they don't or aren't seen to try and rescue a person. Often, a rescuer subconsciously benefits from taking this position. They focus their energy on someone else, which can feel good and get them validation for helping. If they aren't able to help someone, they can say, 'Well, at least I tried', absolving them from guilt. By caring for others, the rescuer can shift focus from themselves onto whoever they are caring for, avoiding people's scrutiny or their own painful internal feelings.

When a rescuer is in relationship with someone who occupies a victim state, they may keep the victim stuck, always needing rescuing. This means that the victim might never emotionally grow or learn to self-soothe. This isn't necessarily a conscious or deliberate result, but it is co-created: the rescuer wants to rescue because it serves their needs, and the victim wants to be recused because it serves theirs. They can trap each other in this cycle for a long time.

The persecutor

The persecutor is also in a co-created relationship, but instead of rescuing, they act like a critical parent, giving out 'tough love' by being strict. They may blame victims for occupying the victim state and criticise rescuers for enabling the victim. It's common for this criticism to be unsolicited, unconstructive, or unachievable. Sexual abuse survivors might hear a persecutor say something like, 'The abuse was years ago. You need to just get on with it and stop moping'. Persecutors often keep control of situations or people by finding faults. This can leave those around them walking on eggshells. People who occupy the victim state can feel controlled or oppressed by persecutors, and this keeps them stuck as victims, never wanting to challenge or push back against the persecutor.

The victim

Victims often feel like they have no power over their lives. They can feel helpless, persecuted, or hopeless. They might say things like, 'Why is it always me?' or 'It always rains when *I* need to go to the shops!' when talking about everyday things. They are at the mercy of life and are often unwilling to take responsibility for the negative things that happen to them. They seek to blame others for their difficult circumstances, like a persecutor, and look to the rescuer to solve problems for them. They can remain stuck in this hopeless place, feeling powerless to change things and unable to take satisfaction or achieve anything.

These different states fuel each other. No one can be a rescuer, persecutor, or victim by themselves; they need another person to enable this type of relationship.

Male survivors who occupy these states

Sexual abuse can often cause male survivors to occupy one of these states.

SURVIVORS AS RESCUERS

The abuse survivor in the rescuer role often fusses and worries about everyone. This may manifest as protectiveness over family, particularly children, or other survivors. In the male survivor recovery groups I run, I have heard many men say a version of 'I've done lots of work on myself. I don't need therapy or support. I want to share what I have learned and help support other male survivors'.

Interestingly, these men are often the first to have flashbacks or bad dreams at the start of the group therapy process. While these symptoms can mean many things, I see them as a sign that, in a room full of survivors sharing stories, the rescuer state might not be powerful enough to keep sexual abuse trauma locked away. Memories start to float up from the survivor's subconscious.

SURVIVORS AS PERSECUTORS

Male survivors who are persecutors can have very black-and-white ideas about justice. They might call for the death penalty for all abusers or chastise other survivors who haven't tried a particular form of therapy. In groups, they are often popular with other survivors; it is a cathartic feeling to hear black-and-white discussions about right and wrong and angry persecutions of abusers. However, survivors in the persecutor role can also become divisive if they persecute a group member or the therapist leading the group. Their overly critical voice can be cathartic to those who need to feel anger towards the world but hurtful to those whom they decide to criticise.

In 2023, I wrote an article about the Drama Triangle for *Therapy Today*. I asked Jack, a survivor, about being in a persecutor state. He told me,

> I just hurt people in my life. If they said to me, 'Look, we love you but you, we know what you've been through, but you can't behave like this', I would ignore them or shout at them or tell them how stupid they were being. Someone made a complaint about me at work for being pushy and angry. This was mad to me, because I always enjoyed work; I liked helping or advising people. I didn't see it as pushy and angry. I almost lost my job, not because they were going to fire me, but because I thought, 'Fuck you! I'm going to leave, then you'll see how stupid you're all being'.[4]
>
> —Jack, white, 57 years old

SURVIVORS AS VICTIMS

Male survivors who take on the victim role can find themselves caught in a painful contradiction. They often feel victimised and are constantly looking for someone to rescue them. They can look for rescuing in relationships, like a supportive friend or a mother figure at work, or more negative influences, such as gang culture, extremist ideologies, or coercive and controlling people. This search may go unnoticed because society often tells men that they can't be victims (eg, *Men should not cry*, *Men should be tough* etc.). Men may feel like no one could possibly understand them while also looking out for someone to rescue them.

This may lead male survivors who occupy the victim state to feel intense shame. They know society expects them to be strong and masculine, and to be a victim is unacceptable. This is extremely difficult for survivors because they can feel shamed by a persecutor who criticises them and also by a rescuer for needing help in the first place. Shame, as much as the persecutor and rescuer, keeps them trapped in this isolated victim state (see Chapter 5, page 82).

Calming Panic Attacks

When to try this: Try this when you feel rising panic. Attempt to do this before a full panic attack takes hold

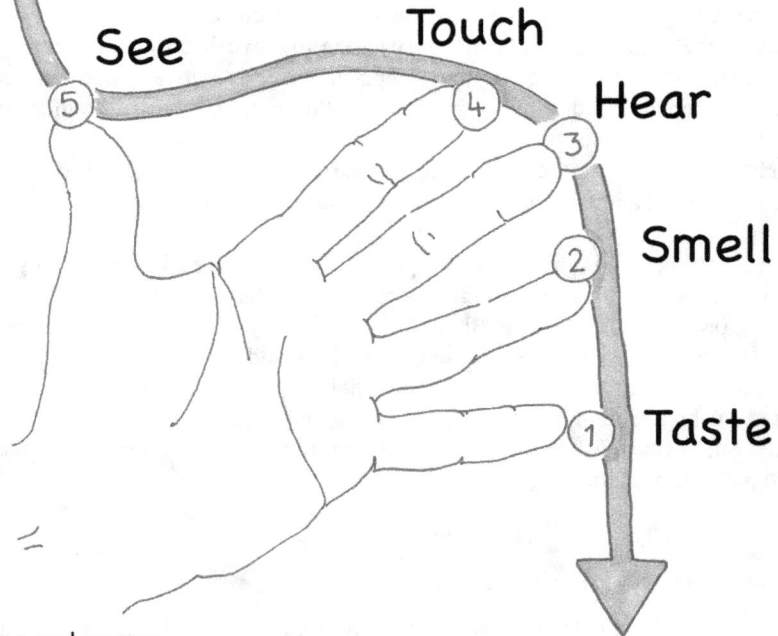

See   Touch   Hear   Smell   Taste

Try and name:

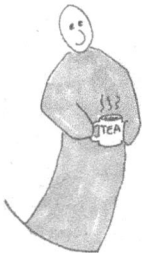

⑤ Five things you can see

④ Four things you can touch

③ Three things you can hear

② Two things you can smell

① One thing you can taste

www.jeremysachs.com @JeremySachs_

For A4 and printable versions of this worksheet, visit www.jeremysachs.com

For A4 and printable versions of this worksheet, visit www.jeremysachs.com

Resources

Trauma Is Really Strange *by Steve Haines*

ISBN: 9781848192935

This is an illustrated comic book that goes into detail about trauma. It isn't specific to certain types of traumatic events, like sexual abuse, but is a good all-around deep dive into the brain and trauma responses.

'Prejudice, social stress, and mental health in lesbian, gay, and bisexual populations: Conceptual issues and research evidence' by Ilan H. Meyer

www.ncbi.nlm.nih.gov

This research paper looks at the experience of minority stress and is free to read from the National Library of Medicine as of July 2024.

A Practical Handbook on Adverse Childhood Experiences (ACEs) Delivering Prevention, Building Resilience and Developing Trauma-Informed Systems: A Resource for Professionals and Organisations *by the WHO*

phwwhocc.co.uk

This is free resource aimed at professionals and charities. However, it gives detailed definitions of ACEs and a broad look at their prevalence in the UK that may interest survivors. Available for free.

Signposting

PTSD UK

www.ptsduk.org

PTSD UK is the only charity in the UK dedicated to raising awareness of PTSD, no matter the trauma that caused it.

Mind

www.mind.org.uk

Local Mind organisations provide various services, including counselling, peer support groups and information on accessing NHS services.

Notes

1 Ilan H. Meyer, 'Prejudice, social stress, and mental health in lesbian, gay, and bisexual populations: Conceptual issues and research evidence', *Psychological Bulletin* 129, no. 5 (September 2003): 674–697. doi: 10.1037/0033-2909.129.5.674.
2 Jiaqi Li, Yu Jin, Shicun Xu, Xianyu Luo, Amanda Wilson, Hui Li, Xiaofeng Wang, Xi Sun, and Yuanyuan Wang, 'Anxiety and depression symptoms among youth survivors of childhood sexual abuse: A network analysis', *BMC Psychology* 11 (September 2023): 278.
3 Stephen B. Karpman, 'Fairy tales and script drama analysis', Group Facilitation: St. Paul, no. 11 (2011): 49–52. https://www.proquest.com/docview/915688199?pq-origsite=gscholar&fromopenview=true&sourcetype=Scholarly%20Journals, accessed 2 August 2024.
4 Jeremy Sachs, 'Escaping the Drama Triangle', *Therapy Today* 34, no. 3 (April 2023): 30.

Chapter 4

Masculinity

How to build a man

Chapter Contents

Not bad enough

Looking back, I realised I had two battles to fight, one was battling the damage of sexual abuse, the second was giving myself permission be impacted by it.

It only happened once as a child. It was a short and confusing violation my child brain couldn't understand and put into the box with everything else that had been going on around me and to me at that time.

As I got older, I seemed to occupy two contradictory spaces. One part of me was paralysed by the idea of sex. I would never ask anyone on a date, never kiss anyone, never make any sort of sexually motivated move. There were women who wanted me to, but I couldn't. I was afraid of somehow victimising them. I needed permission for everything, and at the time, I never met anyone who could give that (or was interested in helping out this painfully shy boy). The second part of me was driven to masturbate. The internet was in its infancy and not everyone had computers. I would risk everything to look at porn, using friend's computers at their parents' house and, when I got old enough, the shop computer where I worked. The shame crushed me every time.

One night in a dazed shameful fog, I felt my abuser's hands on me again. It was a sort of flashback. The memory came flooding back. My skin burned where I could feel his hands had been. I was sick and spent the next three days in bed. I would masturbate, which only confused me more, I hated myself for it.

DOI: 10.4324/9781003423331-4

Coming to terms with these flashbacks and memories and shame was the first battle – eventually it led me to a survivor's support group. I needed to take charge. I wanted a normal relationship, I didn't want to feel shame at masturbating and, if possible, do it less. By the third meeting, other men had shared their stories. I admired them for the bravery, but that sick feeling came back; it only happened once to me, all these men were abused multiple times or in violent ways. I was nothing compared to them. I was an impostor and as soon as these men found out, I'd be kicked out the group. They would spit on me for betraying their trust. So what if a Scout leader had done those things to me, it was hardly bad in comparison.

One meeting I had what felt like a breakdown, although later the guys told me it wasn't nearly as big as it felt. I opened up about my story. They pointed out that it was still horrible, confusing, and shouldn't have happened. The facilitator also pointed out all the other things that happened to me or around me, the violent dad, the divorce, the bullying, the bed-wetting. This was my second battle, acknowledge that my pain was legitimate. I was allowed to take space for my recovery. The guys in the group helped me so much with this. I am so grateful to them.

Adam, 46, Jewish

4.1 How do we define masculinity?

Throughout this book I give examples on the topics included. This helps me think and write about the topics and, hopefully, helps you think about them too. However, I have struggled to do the same thing with the topic of masculinity. Giving examples of masculinity feels reductive because the concept of masculinity is huge. It is sown into the DNA of our society; it is inescapable. This means whatever our identity, it is affected by masculinity. A disabled man may be affected by societal expectations of men's bodies; a Black man may be affected by parts of society with bigoted expectations of Black men. On top of this, masculinity is a fluid concept, making it even harder for me to give concrete examples or provide a solid definition.

To get some sense of this fluidity, imagine we have a time machine. We could travel through time and observe many different incarnations of what it was to be a man throughout history. One fun aspect of masculinity we might see in our time machine is men's historical relationship to high heeled shoes. Did you know that, up until relatively recently, men wore high heels as a symbol of high social status and military prowess? This started in 10th-century Persia. High heels kept cavalry soldier's feet in their stirrups. This was not only practical but demonstrated to the world that men in heels were manly, brave soldiers as well as being wealthy. By the end of the 17th century, this fashion had caught on in Europe, and aristocrats in Germany, Russia, and Spain were all wearing high heels due to their association with success, power, and strength. The style only started to fade around 1730, as women's shoes became more ornate, including the addition of higher heels. Men suddenly didn't want to wear heels due to their new feminisation.

If we took another trip in our time machine, this time to Europe in the Middle Ages, we'd see masculinity defined by family, work, and importantly, the church. This masculinity valued piousness, strong faith, and sexual abstinence outside marriage. Flash forward to Britain during the First World War, and masculinity becomes defined by army conscription propaganda. Aggression became praiseworthy, and patriotism was essential to manliness, as illustrated by the mantra 'For King and Country'. In more recent times, our time machine would show us how capitalism has shaped an individualistic and materialistic concept of masculinity. Money, high-powered jobs, and material objects are all seen as status symbols that define what it is to be 'a successful man'. Our time machine is good at showing us societal ideas of masculinity and how they have changed through history. This is useful because men's views on fashion, sexual relationships, patriotism, and material wealth still affect us today. Acknowledging these ideas' fluidity can help us understand our own relationship to society's views on masculinity.

However, the time machine cannot show us what it is to feel like a man. That is because while society shapes and moulds masculinity, there is also an internal, felt aspect to it. From birth, I have never needed to question whether I am a man. An internal sense of myself, beyond genitalia, tells me I am one. Those men who were assigned female at birth have a similar sense of knowing they are men. The body they were born into, however, may require them to question that sense of masculinity. They may have to go on a journey to establish their relationship with their masculinity, but they nevertheless have an internal, felt sense of being a man. Something inside us, beyond societal expectations and genitals, tells us we are men.

As this chapter progresses, I encourage you to think about your own internal sense of masculinity. Though masculinity gets complicated, particularly for male survivors, your own internal sense of masculinity can help guide you through the abuse. If that sounds daunting, don't worry. The following reflective activity contains ideas on how to start thinking about what masculinity means to you. Keep in mind, you don't need to figure it out all at once. You can save this reflective activity for later or dedicate some time to it before reading the rest of the chapter. This is *your* internal sense of being a man, so it's important not to rush; figuring out what masculinity means to you can be a lifelong project and can change over time because, as we've seen, masculinity is fluid.

Reflective activity

This activity considers three approaches to getting in touch with your authentic, internal sense of masculinity. As you go through these questions, pay attention to how you feel. Do some questions make you feel uncomfortable? Do some make you feel a sense of loss? Are some liberating or even boring? Rather than dismissing these feelings, ask yourself why these questions make you feel this way. Simply striving to understand why some questions about masculinity can make you feel a certain way can be the start to understanding ourselves a little better.

1. Turn *masculinity* plural

Often, masculinity is presented to boys and men as a monolith. It can feel like there is only one version of masculinity, at which you either succeed or fail. I would argue that this sets men up to fail. It is impossible to live up to the narrow and oversimplified ideas of masculinity society offers. It leaves no space for individualism, interpretation, or femininity. In short, it fails all men. It can especially fail men whose authentic self feels far from society's standard, including (but definitely not limited to) stay-at-home dads, disabled, older, gay and trans men, and nonbinary masculine people.

You can combat this by turning *masculinity* into *masculinities*. To do this, think about different men you know and respect. Write down the different ways they express masculinity. This can be behaviour, fashion sense, sexuality, profession, etc.

If you get stuck, famous public figures are a good way to start. For example, you might choose

- Frank Sinatra (Singer)
- Harry Styles (Singer)
- Elliot Page (Actor)
- Freddie Mercury (Singer)
- Pedro Pascal (Actor)
- David Weir (Paralympian)
- Stormzy (Rapper)
- Denzel Washington (Actor)
- Jason Statham (Actor)
- Hozier (Singer/songwriter)
- Ian McKellen (Actor)
- Terry Crews (Actor)
- Rio Ferdinand (Sportsman)
- Dwayne 'The Rock' Johnson (Actor)
- Tom Daley (Olympian)

Feel free to pick your own men or male public figures. Then ask yourself,

- In what ways do these men embody different types of masculinity?
- How do these masculinities differ from each other?
- Are there aspects of these masculinities that make you uncomfortable? If so, why? Have you internalised another person's voice (like a parent or spouse) that says you should/shouldn't like them?
- What parts of their masculinity do you find impressive, fun, or respectable?
- Are there parts of these men's masculinity that you would want to emulate if society let you? Try to pick one thing from each man as examples of different types of masculinity.

The purpose of examining these men and which of their qualities you like or dislike is to recognise that in today's society, many different types of masculinity exist at the same time. It can be useful to examine which types you like, how it feels to think about them, and how that opens up different options for you. These qualities should be authentic aspects of masculinity that you like, rather than qualities that have been chosen for you by other people.

2. Permission

Were there things you were told that you could not do as a child because of your gender? Or things you wanted to do but didn't, knowing someone would disapprove? This can include simple activities such as enjoying particular songs, wearing specific types of clothes, or participating in certain sports or activities. Do you still feel these things are 'not allowed', even as an adult? Sometimes the people who told us we could not do things as children had such power that, even as adults, we hear them police what we are or are not allowed to do as men.

I remember being told as a child that boys didn't make friendship bracelets and men didn't wear jewellery because it was 'poofy'.

This stayed with me well into my thirties, until I bought a friendship bracelet-making kit last year. I was terrible at making them: they came undone, were untidy, and generally a bit rubbish. What is important is that I realised that trying to make them did not compromise my masculinity. Sure, making friendship bracelets was not for me. However, I learned this not because of hypermasculine men in my childhood, but because I simply didn't enjoy it. I also now wear a necklace. It isn't particularly sentimental, but it is a small protest against someone else forcing their ideas of masculinity onto me.

Following is a list of activities that male survivors I have worked with have challenged themselves to do as adults that they previously felt discouraged from doing because of someone else's idea of masculinity. The men were either told directly they could not do these activities or internalised other people's voices preventing them from giving the activities a go. You might be surprised how simple some of these are, but that illustrates other people's power in policing our sense of masculinity and the importance for you as a man to identify our own version.

- Wear nail varnish
- Order an oat flat white coffee instead of a strong black coffee
- Join a yoga class
- Enjoy cheesy pop music
- Feel broody around children
- Order a non-alcoholic drink or a half-pint of beer
- Use moisturiser
- Tell a close friend or family member that they love them
- Admit to being bad at DIY
- Have top surgery
- Ask for parental leave
- Allow themselves to cry in emotional situations or at films
- Say 'I don't know'
- Get pampered at a fancy hairdresser's, get a massage, or take a warm bath with bubbles and candles
- Ask to be 'little spoon' when cuddling
- Wear brightly coloured clothes
- Take a pay cut in order to prioritise job satisfaction over economic success
- Seek out help with the experience of sexual abuse

Can you make a list of things you feel you're not allowed to do because of your gender? This can include things you were specifically told you couldn't do and new things you feel you're not allowed to do.

Once you've written your own list, pick one thing and give yourself permission to give it a go. You don't have to keep doing it; just give yourself permission to do something another person's version of masculinity once discouraged you from doing. Who knows? It might become an activity you want to do regularly or, like my friendship bracelets, simply a one-off experience. Either way, you will be building an authentic relationship with your own personal version of masculinity.

3. Journaling

Men are seldom asked how they feel or allowed space to reflect on emotions. Many versions of masculinity leave no space for complex or varied emotions. Men are often told they are 'logical' rather than emotional. However, this does not mean they don't have emotions, simply that they are not allowed to voice or understand their emotions and, therefore, lack practice at recognising them.

Writing a journal or diary is not for everyone. For people who struggle to write due to neurodiversity, difficulty with spelling, sentence structure, and grammar, or simply translating thoughts on to paper, journaling can be a big and overwhelming task. Some men won't know where to start, while others will simply find it doesn't work for them.

Even if journaling doesn't feel like something you'd be good at, a gentle challenge is to spend two to twenty minutes asking yourself how you feel and making a note of it in whatever way works for you. Taking time to regularly identify how you feel can be a powerful tool in getting to know your own sense of masculinity. After doing it for a while, you might see what that's like to share some of those feelings with a friend you trust. For help starting, try to identify some of your feelings on the Emotion Wheel on page 256.

Today's Western culture offers many diverse and broad concepts of masculinity. More than ever, we see versions of masculinity in mainstream culture that would have been unimaginable 50 years ago, from the UK parliament being the 'gayest in the world'[1] to male US rappers painting their nails and featuring in British Vogue magazine.[2] However, this does not make masculinity simpler. In fact, the variety can make masculinity feel more confusing and contradictory. Men must be strong and men must be vulnerable. Men must be the financial provider and men must be available in the home. Men should protect and men should let their defences down. Men can be gay as long as they don't 'act gay'.

For male survivors of sexual abuse, these contradictory ideas can be paralysing. I speak to many men who tell me they would encourage all survivors to call a helpline and share their feelings with friends, while at the same time telling me it is impossible for them to take their own advice and ask for help. When I ask why, they answer with 'I don't know' or tell me their pain is 'not that bad'. While more expressive ways to embrace masculinity are more acceptable in more parts of the world than ever before, many of the problematic expectations on men still exist. Some of these older ideas may not be inherently harmful, but they can quickly make men's relationships with the world, their loved ones, and themselves hard to navigate – especially as survivors.

4.2   Toxic masculinity: When masculinity does harm

While definitions of masculinity vary between cultures and times in history, studies tell us there are common traits, particularly in Western cultures. Thompson and Pleck's 1986 paper 'The structure of male role norms'[3] analyses social norms among college men and their relation to women. The paper's definition of masculinity can be briefly summarised as follows:

- **Toughness.** Men should be physically strong, emotionally callous and aggressive.
- **Antifemininity.** Men should reject anything traditionally feminine or emotional and helping behaviour.
- **Power.** Men should work towards attaining both social and financial power and independence, fostering others' respect.

These traits associated with masculinity can make being a man lonely. This version of masculinity is defined by a rejection of femininity and characterised by conflicts for dominance, whether in terms of money, physical strength, or social status. Despite numerous studies on masculinity since the 1980s, the traits identified by researchers like Thompson and Pleck still resonate today, highlighting the enduring struggle men face in navigating their relationship with these norms.

In the UK, Thompson and Pleck's masculine traits are encapsulated in the 'hard man' archetype. This tough, resilient figure is familiar across different cultures, each with its own version. The hard man is celebrated and glorified, particularly in places like South London and Glasgow, where I grew up and live now respectively. I've seen the hard man archetype take on almost mythical proportions in these environments, to the extent that even being associated with these locations confers a sense of masculine credibility. For example, the opening line in rapper Dave's track 'Streatham' – 'Look, I grew up in Streatham' – immediately sets a tone signalling the violent, masculine environment that shaped him. Similarly, the hard man is deeply ingrained in Scottish identity, particularly in the city of Glasgow. You may have similar examples of this in the area where you live.

The trouble with the hard man archetype is that it's a fantasy. Striving to embody that fantasy sets men up for failure, with devastating consequences for individuals, families, and communities. In 2005, the WHO named Glasgow the murder capital of Europe,[4] highlighting the intersection of poverty, substance abuse, unemployment, and problematic masculinity in contributing to this grim statistic.

In recent years, there's been an attempt to rebrand problematic masculine archetypes with terms like 'alpha male', positioned as modern, updated versions of the hard man. Despite the rebranding, however, these archetypes remain harmful. The concept of the alpha male, originally derived from observation of wolf packs, is now understood to be outdated even in the context of wolves:

> It turns out that this is a myth, and in recent years wildlife biologists have largely dropped the term 'alpha'. In the wild, researchers have found that most wolf packs are simply families, led by a breeding pair, and bloody duels for supremacy are rare.[5]

When we search the internet for a definition of the human alpha male, things get confusing quickly. The results are full of articles like 'Nine signs you're an alpha male', along with products like vitamin supplements specifically targeted at 'alpha men'. *Harvard Business Review* will tell you that 70 per cent of senior executives are alpha men who 'aren't happy unless they're the top dogs'. According to the same article, they've 'found top women rarely if ever match the complete alpha profile'.[6] Looking through these articles, you'll find lots of opinions and pseudoscientific terms, but very little in the way of actual behavioural or social science. Dig a little deeper, and you'll find dating advice from alpha men to men who *want* to be alpha. It quickly becomes misogynistic, aggressive and manipulative. Some of it is chilling.

It can be difficult to distinguish problematic masculine traits from healthy expressions of masculinity. This is because in much of society, the hard man archetype and alpha male culture often incorporate traditionally masculine traits that are not harmful. I want to be clear to men reading this who want to identify with traditional masculine traits that this is not a bad thing. Strength, reliability, and protectiveness are all positive things that are good to aspire to as individual traits. However, it becomes problematic when society tells men that traditional masculine traits are the only option, even at the cost of their mental health and relationships and other people's wellbeing. This is what we might call *toxic masculinity*.

Toxic masculinity is a term originally used in the 1980s by the mythopoetic men's movement, which believed that society no longer allowed men to express traditionally masculine behaviours; men couldn't act on their 'manliness'. The moment created spaces where men could meet and take part rituals, storytelling, and drumming. Since then, the term *toxic masculinity* has evolved and is used in social, feminist, and gender studies.

I define toxic masculinity as a collection of exaggerated behaviours and attitudes that are considered masculine and are encouraged and supported by society. They are behaviours or attitudes that consider extreme individualism and lack of empathy as virtues while glorifying aggression, harmful capitalism, and working to assert dominance over women and femininity, queerness, people from minority backgrounds, and disabled people. Toxic masculinity is an unattainable set of principles and expectations of men to which people of all genders can be susceptible and that perpetuates harm to boys, teens, men, and all those they come into contact with, directly or indirectly.

Toxic masculinity does not tolerate those who are physically weak, gay, fat, disabled, poor. It does not allow men to prioritise family over career, be sensitive, age beyond their thirties, or be in touch with emotions. It cannot comprehend men as victims of any type of crime or abuse. Toxic masculinity allows for only one way to be a man: strong, independent and dominant. The power of toxic masculinity is that it is embedded in a society that tells men how to be. Films, children's toys, social media, high-street brands, and family members of all genders can all be indoctrinated, directing men on how to think and behave. It has also embedded itself inside men's minds, opening a path for them to tell themselves they are weak or not 'man enough' whenever they feel insecure or anxious – the perfect echo chamber for shame and self-loathing.

I argue that toxic masculinity is a natural enemy of all male survivors of sexual abuse. It stops us acknowledging the damage of abuse and prevents us recovering and living authentic lives. It also discourages people from supporting, believing, or respecting us.

4.3   Myths and stigma internalised by survivors

When men do not meet the expectations set in toxic masculinity, they are belittled or punished. A man seeking help by disclosing a rape is an easy target for punishment. Often, this punishment comes in the form of weaponised myths and stigma about sexual abuse, as in saying, 'Men can't be raped!' This is hugely damaging to men and society as a whole. Myths and stigma enable perpetrators to continue harming children, teens and adults. They also prevent survivors from getting support. Before long, survivors can start to internalise these myths and stigma. Without anyone to validate their experience, some survivors can believe that they are in some way at fault for being abused or raped. Others may diminish their experiences, as in, *I need to 'man up'!* Men often have two internal voices. One is an authentic voice that knows they are not to blame for what happened. The other is the voice of toxic masculinity, which keeps the myths and stigma alive by telling them they are to blame for the abuse or they should just get on with it and stop being weak.

Following is a list of 16 myths and stigma that toxic masculinity helps to fuel. All of them protect perpetrators and harm survivors, preventing them from getting help and living a more authentic life.

1.   Transgender men are confused about their gender because of childhood sexual abuse

This myth is rooted in transphobia, misunderstands gender dysphoria, and can be psychologically damaging to survivors of sexual assault and the trans community. There is also zero scientific evidence behind this myth. Sadly, some healthcare professionals perpetuate this myth by denying trans patients access to gender reassignment clinics because they believe sexual abuse has influenced the patient's decision to seek medical support in transitioning. Therapists can also perpetuate this myth by pathologising trans identity. Trans people experience this not only in healthcare. Often friends and family use this myth in attempt to make sense of a trans person's identity. They may not mean harm with this belief, but they are nevertheless perpetuating a damaging believe about trans people and trans survivors.

2. Being sexually abused by a man makes male survivors gay

This myth is not correct. However you define your sexuality, being sexually abused by any gender doesn't inform your sexual orientation. Yet many people believe this. As with the transphobia in the previous myth, this myth is rooted in homophobia and implies being gay is a choice or unnatural. Combined with the shame and self-loathing caused by sexual abuse, this myth can make some gay men believe that surviving sexual abuse by another man made them gay. This can be particularly powerful if the survivor grew up in a family or community where being gay is considered bad or sinful. The survivor may use this form of internalised homophobia to punish themselves or other gay people.

Straight men are also affected by this myth. Some men live in fear of appearing gay due to toxic expectations on heterosexual people. They may refuse to seek help in case someone 'accuses' them of being gay or doing 'gay activities'. This fear of appearing homosexual is particularly uncomfortable and damaging. It is harmful on multiple fronts, perpetuating homophobia while also preventing men from seeking help.

3. Gay men are paedophiles

This is an extremely old myth that doesn't just affect sexual abuse survivors, but LGBTQIA+ people in general. It implies that people who are not heterosexual are sexually deviant, abusive, and untrustworthy around children.

4. Men who were sexually abused go on to sexually abuse others

Unlike the previous myth – *Gay men are paedophiles* – this myth specifically targets survivors. It is a complicated and triggering myth for many men. The vast majority of survivors do not abuse others. In fact, most men who are abused develop a strong sense of social justice and support others, either formally through work and volunteering or informally through being a good friend and confidant.

I have heard speakers at conferences on sexual abuse announce that this myth is 100 per cent untrue. However, I believe this issue has more nuance. A small minority of people who have been abused will harm others. This harm can be violence, emotional neglect, child-on-child abuse, other forms of abuse, and yes, sexual harm. Some survivors may do this as a child or teenager to another child or teenager, replicating what has been done to them. Others, for complex and painful reasons, may seek to sexually harm others in adulthood.

Unfortunately, the myth that all or most men who are abused grow up to abuse others is so damaging to men that conversations about survivors who do harm others are shut down immediately by professionals and survivors alike. They do this to protect the vast majority of male survivors from stigma and bigotry, but they do so at the cost of any conversation that may improve this marginalised issue.

Often missing is a look at the bigger picture. If a man was sexually abused, he is likely to have faced many other abuses and challenges (see Chapter 3, page 52, for ACEs). This may include physical abuse, food insecurity, emotional neglect, or a sadistic parent or teacher. It is likely that a combination of factors and adverse early experiences leads men to sexually violent or abusive behaviour rather than any one experience of sexual abuse. Being sexually abused does not predetermine abuse of others. An expression often used by scientists and mathematicians sums this up well: correlation is not causation. Just because a *very* small number of survivors do sexual harm to others doesn't mean that the experience of sexual abuse caused them to do so.

The truth is that many male survivors fear harming others – a fear that can become a prison they struggle to escape from. Male survivors often become extremely distressed worrying about whether they will go on to do harm. This can cause extreme isolation and self-disgust. They can avoid dating, family, or any situation where children may be present. This is not because they want to abuse children, but because the damage of their own abuse was so profound, that any risk of doing any harm to others is too dangerous for them psychologically. However, a small minority of men do commit harm, and while they are also survivors of sexual abuse, this experience alone is unlikely to be the single reason they abuse others.

5. If men engage in risky behaviour like chemsex parties or causal hook-ups, they are 'asking for it'

Agreeing to attend a chemsex party (a place where drugs are taken in order to have sex, see Chapter 7, page 138), using hookup apps or meeting for casual sex does not mean you are agreeing to sex or any other activity someone else wants to do. Being present in an environment where sex happens or where there is an expectation of sex is not the same as giving consent. Even in these environments, any sexual activity that you do not want or do not consent to is assault.

6. Sexual abuse is only a problem for gay men

Sexual abuse, especially in adulthood, is often labelled as a 'gay problem'. This is problematic on many levels. It is homophobic because it singles out gay men, making a judgement about gay culture and gay experiences while marginalising the experiences of men with different identities. There are theories about the correlation between gayness and the experience of sexual abuse (see Chapter 7, page 130), but labelling something a 'gay problem' is diminishing, discriminatory, and inaccurate.

7. Men can't be sexually abused by women

Women perpetrate sexual abuse. This can be hard for many to imagine. Some can't believe a man could be victimised by the 'the weaker sex'; others can't believe a woman, who 'should be' caring and motherly, could commit such harm. These attitudes are problematic for survivors, women, and society as a whole, because the truth is that women are just as capable of committing harm as men. Data on the proportion of female perpetrators is hard to find, in part because the additional shame attached to being abused by a woman may prevent men from coming forward (see Chapter 5, page 96). However, based on my own anecdotal experience, each group of 12 I run has around one or two male survivors of abuse by a woman – anyone from mothers and teachers to wives, partners, friends, and colleagues.

8. Sexual abuse doesn't happen in Black communities

Some Black men report that, within certain parts of their community, sexual abuse is seen as an issue that only affects non-Black people. This belief, coupled with a cultural attitude that people should 'just get on with it' rather than 'dwelling on their problems', can be isolating and make it hard for Black survivors to find spaces that can fully support them. As Tarana Burke, an African American activist and the founder of the #MeToo movement, said, '[s]exual violence knows no race, class, or gender. It can happen to anyone, anywhere. The idea that it doesn't happen in our community is one of the biggest fallacies'.[7] Due in part to this myth, Black people, along with people from other minority backgrounds, can experience challenges when finding formal help. Disadvantages from medical racism to lack of representation in therapeutic services mean that some people never feel fully seen as a survivor and as a person of colour.

9. Disabled men should consider themselves lucky

People often make a judgement about the sexual capital of disabled people. These men may be viewed as non-sexual, an attitude that can be communicated explicitly or through a lack of representation. This attitude is harmful and problematic, suggesting that these men should not feel sexual desire or have authentic Sexual Selves. It also means that when a disabled man is sexually abused, many people will dismiss or disbelieve it or not take it seriously. Some men have shared with me that they've been told they are 'lucky' to have had any sexual contact, even if that contact comes without their consent. The marginalisation of men who are seen as non-sexual, along with the myth that men welcome any sexual contact, leaves these men vulnerable to perpetrators and abuse.

Adding further complexity, the identifier 'disabled' is a broad one that seldom reflects the diversity, identity, and experiences of all disabled people. For example, many men with disabilities are able to consent to sexual contact; however, some men with disabilities, such as learning disabilities, may not have capacity to consent to sex. In some cases, they may communicate a desire for sex, but this is distinct from demonstration of capacity to consent. A capacity assessment or even a court of protection might be needed to determine a learning-disabled person's capacity to consent. Additionally, some disabled men may have communication challenges that make them unable to identify or talk about abuse they experience. People often neglect these cases' nuance, so scared of the complexities and difficulties of the issue that they willingly ignore abuse or signs of abuse in people under their care. There is also a lack of platforms for disabled men to voice their experiences within the dialogue about sex and abuse. This lack of platform not only allows myths and stigma to continue diminishing these men, but it also creates an environment where power and sexual abuses go unnoticed or are not taken seriously.

10. If you get aroused or orgasm, then you must have enjoyed it

Getting an erection, being aroused, and ejaculating or orgasming have nothing to do with consent and do not mean you enjoyed nonconsensual sexual contact. When physically stimulated in a particular way, the nerve endings in our bodies respond whether we consent or not. Physical arousal and feelings that are physically pleasant do not equal enjoyment, consent, or that a survivor 'wanted it'.

11. Men always want sex and therefore cannot be sexually abused

There is a common belief that men always want sex and therefore must desire any sexual attention. This untrue myth is particularly toxic, as it removes men's agency, sense of self and Sexual Self completely from sexual encounters.

Men's identity and common stereotypes can complicate this even more. Some groups of men – for instance, Black men – are often fetishised, while other racial groups – such as Asian men – are often feminised. Harmful stereotypes and racialised myths like these make it easier for people to dismiss these men or minimise their experiences. It can also feed into men's own low self-worth and shame or create internalised stigma towards their own gender and race (for more on the Sexual Self, see Chapter 7, page 130).

12.   In some situations, survivors are partly to blame

Nonconsensual sex is not your fault. It is a crime and entirely the responsibly of the perpetrator. Often, people can blame survivors for the way they dress, how much they drink, how high they get, or whether they go home with someone. This is victim blaming. Some perpetrators, particularly in cases of childhood, teenage, or domestic abuse, can make survivors believe that they want sex or sexual contact. They can create an environment where they so control the victim that the victim instigates sexual contact. This is manipulation and a type of grooming.

This myth can also become difficult when both the survivor and perpetrator are children. Abuse among children is often the result of one child's premature sexualisation, often through abuse or early exposure to pornography. Due to the perpetrator's young age, people can assume some grey area exists or that the abuse must not be too bad.

It is worth me repeating: *it was not your fault.* The responsibility for what happened lies directly with the perpetrator. It is not about your actions before the assault. The perpetrator made a choice, and they committed a crime.

13.   You need to forgive the perpetrator

People will feel different ways about this. Some survivors need to find forgiveness towards their perpetrator. Others wish only the worst things imaginable for them. I believe that you don't have to forgive anybody. You are the one who was sexually abused, and you get to decide how to feel towards the perpetrator and anyone who failed to protect you. If it feels useful to work towards forgiveness, then absolutely do this. However, it is your right to decide how you feel and what helps you heal. If forgiveness of the perpetrator is not part of that journey, that is okay (see Chapter 11, page 211).

14.   It was a long time ago; you should move on

Sexual abuse is like an explosion at the core of who we are, and the impact of abuse can still be felt many years later. Many male survivors say that the most significant impact wasn't the act of sexual abuse itself (horrific as it was), but the damage it did to their sense of self and their relationships with others. *Moving on* is a vague term that implies you should forget what happened to you, but your history is your history and cannot be forgotten. What *can* happen is that you integrate the abuse into the story of your life in a way that gives you control and stops the damaging impact.

15.   Online sexual abuse isn't that bad

The term *online sexual abuse* can cover a variety of experiences, from the exploitation of children and young people on the internet to revenge porn (see Chapter 1, page 15). While online sexual abuse may not include a physical attack, it can still have a devastating impact. Often, it involves being groomed or tricked into a trusting relationship, only for trust to be broken or the relationship to be fake. It can have a deep and disturbing impact on someone's life. It is often shaming and humiliating and used to exercise power over someone. Nevertheless, online sexual abuse is often dismissed as something people should 'get over', and the damage is often downplayed or misunderstood. Revenge porn (or threatening someone with revenge porn) only became illegal in the UK in 2015, and we have a long way to go on taking this form of abuse seriously.

16.   *You should report it*

For some survivors, reporting can help them regain a sense of power while for others, it risks digging up some of the worst experiences of their lives. It also comes with no guarantees of a conviction. Reporting to the police can be a long and pain-ful process that ends without justice. In some cases, the police can also retraumatise survivors. Different communities are treated differently by police, and depending on your identity, you might not feel safe reporting. You might decide to report the abuse to the police, or you might decide that wouldn't be helpful for you. In some cases, it may not be possible; the perpetrator may be dead, in another country, or unknown to you. Reporting is your decision to make, and no one else has the right to pressure you either way.

As I write the last few lines of this chapter, I'm struck by how overwhelming this topic is. I don't mind sharing this has been one of the hardest chapters to write. I was brought up in an environment where ideas about masculinity were extremely narrow and mixed with shame and aggression. Writing this chapter has made me reflect on my early experiences of masculinity and question many of my beliefs about men and masculinity today. I've swung between anger, shame, and numb-ness in the process of putting these thoughts in words. I'm sharing this because I suspect that if I've had a hard time writing it, it may also have been hard for you to read.

From the moment we're born, our society bombards us with messages about what it means to be a man and how men should behave. These messages deeply influence our internal and external perceptions of ourselves. Then comes along sexual abuse that smashes apart our world and our view of ourselves as men.

As men and survivors who have already faced so much, we can feel pressure to find quick solutions to our problems or pain. However, as we have seen, mas-culinity is not any one fixed thing. It evolves throughout our lives and can mean different things to us at different times. Give yourself permission to explore and redefine your understanding of masculinity at your own pace. Use the tools in this book or reach out to a friend or loved one. I believe that masculinity is absolutely more complex than the narrow vision society dictates, and our masculinity and our sense of it is much more than the impact of sexual abuse.

Ways to Calm Anxiety

1 — Put your hands in cold water.

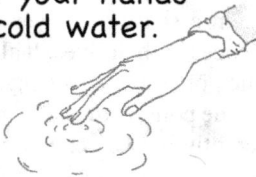

2 — Use breathing exercises, like the Square Breathing in this book.

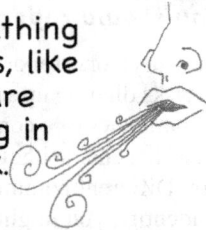

3 — Eat strong flavoured sweets and focus on the taste and sensation.

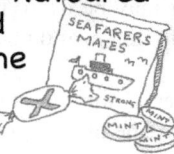

SEAFARERS MATES

STRONG MINT MINT

4 — Find a smell you enjoy, and if you feel the need to ground yourself, take some deep sniffs of the smell.

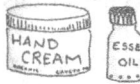

HAND CREAM   ESSE OIL

5 — Change your environment—this could be going into a different room or a trip to the local park.

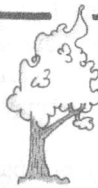

6 — Move your body, for example: stretches in your chair, yoga, or swimming.

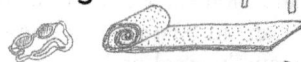

When to try these: It is best to try and calm anxiety before you reach crisis point. Practise doing one of these each time something feels stressful. This way when anxiety starts to build, you will have practised something that helps you calm stressful feelings.

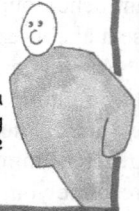

www.jeremysachs.com @JeremySachs_

For A4 and printable versions of this worksheet, visit www.jeremysachs.com

For A4 and printable versions of this worksheet, visit www.jeremysachs.com

Resources

Mask Off: Masculinity Redefined *by J. J. Bola*

This book exposes masculinity as a performance into which men are socially conditioned. Using examples of non-Western cultural traditions, music and sport, it shines light on historical narratives around manhood, debunking popular myths along the way.

Sons and Others: On Loving Male Survivors *by Tanaka Mhishi*

ISBN: 9781912489640

Sons and Others is a book that challenges misconceptions and misrepresentations of sexual violence against men across media and the broader society. It offers a new way of seeing and understanding these men in our lives, asking how the violence they experience affects us all.

Signposting

Future Men

https://futuremen.org

This is a multi-award-winning specialist charity that supports boys and men along the path to becoming dynamic future men.

Andy's Man Club

http://andysmanclub.co.uk

This is a men's suicide prevention charity, offering free-to-attend peer-to-peer support groups across the United Kingdom and online.

Notes

1 Andrew Reynolds, 'The UK's parliament is still the gayest in the world after 2019 election', The Pink News, 13 December 2019. www.thepinknews.com/2019/12/13/uk-gay-parliament-world-2019-general-election-snp-conservatives-labour-lgbt, accessed 2 August 2024.
2 Hannah Coates, 'This autumn, nail inspiration comes from the guys', *Vogue*, 4 October 2019. www.vogue.co.uk/beauty/article/nail-inspiration-from-boys-asap-rocky, accessed 2 August 2024.
3 Edward H. Thompson and Joseph H. Pleck, 'The structure of male role norms', *American Behavioral Scientist* 29, no. 5 (May/June 1986): 531–533.

4   Gerard Seenan, 'Scotland has second highest murder rate in Europe', *The Guardian*, updated 25 September 2005. www.theguardian.com/uk/2005/sep/26/ukcrime.scotland, accessed 2 August 2024.

5   Stephanie Pappas, 'Is the alpha wolf idea a myth?', *Scientific American*, 28 February 2023.   www.scientificamerican.com/article/is-the-alpha-wolf-idea-a-myth/#:~:text= But%20it%20turns%20out%20that,duels%20for%20supremacy%20are%20rare, accessed 2 August 2024.

6   Kate Ludeman and Eddie Erlandson, 'Coaching the Alpha Male', *Harvard Business Review*, May 2004. https://hbr.org/2004/05/coaching-the-alpha-male.

7   Tarana Burke, '#MeToo was started for black and brown women and girls. They're still being ignored', *Washington Post*, 9 November 2017. www.washingtonpost.com/news/ post-nation/wp/2017/11/09/the-waitress-who-works-in-the-diner-needs-to-know-that- the-issue-of -sexual-harassment-is-about-her-too, accessed 2 August 2024.

Chapter 5

The stomach-dissolving experience of shame

Chapter Contents

Shame

I have spent most of my life carrying a dirty little secret. I have been guilty of something awful. The guilt and shame have been sitting at the back of my mind since 1981 and have always reminded me that I am a bad person, soiled, unclean. A constant nagging at the back of my mind: *You are damaged goods*. Despite a successful career in software and, more recently, finance, I knew that if the truth came out, my acquaintances would abandon me. I have avoided close friendships. Indeed, I don't have friends at all. I am unable to call anyone a friend. I know that I could easily taint anybody that gets close to me. That said, I am married and dearly love my wife. However, intimate contact is difficult, and sex has been impossible for me.

Mid-1990s

In the mid-90s, I am driving home from Oxford listening to Radio 4, where a girl is discussing how she feels after being a victim of rape. Her description is of being unclean, of being dirty, of being unable to wash the violation away, of sensing that nobody would believe her. I find myself in tears and must pull the car over into a lay-by. I am feeling her pain, not just in my imagination but in my memory, I have felt those feelings in the past, in my own experience, but pushed the memory away. A conflict arises from this memory. I am a man; my abuser was an older woman. But men don't get raped by women. It cannot happen. I cannot have been assaulted by this woman. If I share this

DOI: 10.4324/9781003423331-5

with anybody, I will be told that I should consider myself lucky. It was a rite of passage. So why, *why* am I feeling so wretched? I am telling myself that it did not happen. As a male member of society, I would not, could not, accept what I knew to be the truth. This is my dirty little secret: I have been soiled and damaged by the events of 1981 and have been carrying a loathing for myself since then. For allowing it to happen. It is entirely my fault. I hate myself.

A little earlier than this, a visit from an acquaintance I knew at the time of the abuse caught me unawares. I had completely forgotten or pushed away to the back of my mind the fact that he had been present the evening that the 'event' took place. He remarked on the fact that we had been lads and what good times we had had: 'Remember that night...?' It was a devastating blow. It felt like he had physically punched me. The memories were suddenly out. His recollection of what happened clearly differed from mine. The feeling of unwholesomeness was back, and I struggled to push it, and my shame and guilt, back to the place from where it had escaped. I wanted to vomit. I had to get that man out of my house. As long as he was there, I was in a state of panic.

The radio and the visit caused me to look back at my life and memories. More importantly for me, to justify why I felt my memories were lies. I needed to make excuses. I needed to prove to myself that my memories were false. I became quite adept at doing this. Unfortunately, the good memories got filed in my mind as false, as well as the bad ones. What happened to me?

Early 1980s

In 1981, I had dropped out of university and was in a vulnerable state. I had found work for a national chain of shops but hated the antisocial hours, which involved 12 or more hours a day, seven days a week. A family friend, David (not his real name), suggested that I go and work with him for a small insurance company. It wasn't a job I particularly wanted, but he assured me that I would be good at it, and I was sold on the idea if only to escape the retail job. On starting, I was introduced to a work colleague – a woman, Catherine (not her real name) – and over a very short period of weeks, I was rapidly promoted to a more senior position – much more senior than I would have expected as an inexperienced 20-year-old.

Catherine, a woman older than me by some years, was very attentive. She seemed very interested in me. She was fun to be with, exotic, even sexy, although decidedly not my type. She was keen to entertain me, introduce me to her friends, even show me off to some of them. I never asked why. Soon parties and other entertainment were on offer; it was at these that I was shown the *real* world. I was brought up as a Catholic and attended a convent school. I was now shown that the world I had been brought up in was a lie promoted by the church, by my parents. The real world was about sex. Over the course of weeks and months, it became obvious sex was everywhere. Everybody I was introduced to was having frequent sex. With each other, with other partners. This became my only real world.

I distanced myself from family from friends, who I now believed to be liars who had taught me that the world was something different from the reality. As I came to understand the world around me, it became obvious that David and Catherine were not just work colleagues. They were sexual partners, lovers. They would openly discuss me together. I cannot say which of them said it. My memory is Catherine, but it was explained to me that I was to be *her* virgin. She had never fucked a virgin. That was my destiny. I cannot explain why I was not able to run, to escape. I knew that I did not want to lose my virginity in this place to this woman. However, there felt like no one to run to, no place to go from this reality. The pressure to have intercourse with Catherine grew until I was told that the only way this pressure would go away was to agree to sex. It was, after all, 'perfectly normal' and was the only option. One evening, around a friend's house, I finally realised that I had no option.

The immediate aftermath was escape, run home, shower, wash away the guilt of what I had done. But it clung, adhered to every crevice, despite letting the water run until it was cold. I could not wash this 'thing' away. I felt violated, that I had let myself down. I developed an itch, a soreness that began in the hours following. That itch still came back regularly. The itch required me to attend the 'special clinic' which, at the time, was also a degrading experience, emphasising my shame at what I had done. Catherine was gone, no longer interested. My purpose served, I was discarded.

2020

Forty years after the event, a flare-up of the itch caused me seek help. A trip to the nearest genitourinary clinic resulted in being told I hadn't picked up a STD; I just had a urinary tract infection. More to the point, I had never had an STD. Apparently, I should have been told that 40 years earlier. I was referred for counselling, the thought of which terrified me. I knew that the counselling would prove to me just how everything was my own fault. In my mind, counselling was going to justify my fears. However, the counselling has helped me learn how I was groomed by David and Catherine and to explore my feelings and memories. After 40 years of bottling everything up, the relief of having somebody to share my feelings with, somebody who does not judge, has been life-changing.

TDM, cisgender man, raised Roman Catholic

5.1   What is shame?

I remember my therapist once saying, 'It is impossible to have an authentic conversation about shame without feeling shame yourself'. During this therapy session, my story had made my therapist connect with his own shame. We were talking about a time I was shamed 24 years earlier, as a child. Shame doesn't respect time and space. In this case, my childhood shame had time-travelled from back then to the present day. It felt like it had contaminated my adult self, my therapy, and my therapist. That is how strong shame is: it can jump from person to person simply at its mention.

In recovery groups, an expression used to define shame is 'To feel guilt is to feel like you have done something bad; to feel shame is to feel like you are bad'. This expression is useful because *guilt* and *shame* are used interchangeably. It can be hard to know the difference. As survivors seek to undo the damage of sexual abuse, they often feel caught between the two emotions. As we will examine later, sexual abuse can create shame in the survivor. A survivor can feel shame over an abuse that they are not responsible for. This can be the tip of the iceberg for some people, as shame can affect all aspects of a person's identity. Someone can be ashamed of their sexuality, masculinity, gender, disability, or heritage. This can get tangled up in the shame of surviving sexual abuse. Understanding the difference between guilt and shame is a useful step towards understanding some of the painful feelings and behaviours it can cause.

Guilt is like shame in many ways. Guilt is a feeling of regret or sadness about a past action or experience that has caused harm or potential harm to someone. We can also experience it if our actions feel like they break a social code, ethical value, or expectation we have of ourselves. Guilt can fuel social anxiety and low self-esteem. It is difficult to sit with and can cause internal struggle. However, what it does *not* do is feel dangerous and activate a trauma-like response in our bodies – unlike shame.

Shame can make us feel like we are bad on a molecular level, that every cell in our body is wrong. Our stomachs dissolve, and we are left alone in our wrongness, knowing we are bad at our core. This can feel extremely disturbing for survivors – so disturbing, in fact, that it can feel like we are in real danger. Being shamed can send survivors into a trauma response (see page 28 for trauma responses). Some may dissociate; others might have a panic attack or fly into a rage.

Responses to shame can be all-consuming and hard to think about clearly. Cognitive-behavioural therapy (CBT) can provide a useful framework for demystifying feelings of shame and exploring the different parts of us that get activated in reaction to it. CBT is a common type of talking therapy in the UK, especially in the NHS. It looks at how your thoughts, feelings, physical sensations, and actions are connected. CBT helps you understand and break negative cycles of thinking and feeling. Its aim is to show how to deal with problems in a more positive way by breaking them into smaller, more manageable parts. By changing negative patterns,

CBT hopes to improve how clients feel. It is used to treat a range of issues, from eating and personality disorders to PTSD and phobias.

Following is what's called a *cognitive model*, which can be used to slow down the domino effect that shame can activate. It attempts to break down each piece of a situation separately and can apply to shame activated in different situations we find ourselves in: work, with family, out and about, or when we are alone. Try breaking down a shame response in these three stages:

- **Situation.** Set the scene as objectively as possible. What happened to activate your shame? Where were you and who was involved? Think about the practical details of the circumstances that started your shame response.
- **Automatic thoughts.** What were the first thoughts that ran through your mind? This may be one loud thought or several thoughts that blend into one. (These can be a little tricky to identify, so if it is easier, you may want to move onto reactions and come back to this afterwards).
- **Reactions.** CBT is interested in three different kinds of reactions:
  1. **Emotional.** What feelings did you notice having?
  2. **Bodily (physically).** What did you notice physically (for example, feeling hot in the face)?
  3. **Behavioural.** What did you do or what action did you take?

What follows is an everyday example of how someone who is shame-prone might feel shamed at work using CBT classifications.

Situation. Imagine a person arriving at work. They are on time and sit down at their desk to start the day. They make eye contact with their line manager, who then walks over, saying, 'This afternoon, can we have a word?'

For some who are not shame-prone, this may be fine. They will get on with their day and not think twice about what their line manager wants. However, someone who is shame-prone may experience this differently. It might send them into a spiral of familiar and shame-provoked automatic thoughts about themselves.

Automatic thoughts. The shame-provoked automatic thoughts may be

- What have I done wrong?
- I'm so stupid, everyone else in the office is good at their job and I'm not.
- My line manager has finally found out I'm a fraud.

Once this shame-prone person has an automatic thought, they will have a reaction to it. This reaction is likely to present itself emotionally, bodily (or physically), and behaviourally.

Reaction. Emotionally, the shame-prone person may be emotionally angry at their line manager as well as themselves. Their bodily reaction might be to feel hot or start sweating, and behaviourally, they may reach for a cigarette to attempt soothing.

The following list includes various emotional, bodily, and behavioural reactions to shame. A shame-prone person may experience any number of these. While shame is universal and most of us will experience it at some point, it is also deeply personal. Each person will respond to it differently, and how you respond may not be listed here. Consider identifying your own shame reactions in the worksheet on page 89.

Emotional

- **Anger and rage.** A survivor who is shamed can feel instantly angry. This anger can explode outward, aimed at anything or anyone, including loved ones or precious belongings. The anger can also be aimed internally; survivors can be rage-filled at ourselves. Anger can build up, as well. We can feel anger about something and hold onto it over a period of time. Eventually this anger gets released and can be aimed at something or someone that has nothing to do with the shaming incident.
- **Anxiety.** Being shame-prone can create a feeling of unease. Survivors can feel anxiety that prevents us from acting or thinking clearly. This can feel frightening or confusing.
- **Feeling lost.** Shame can alter our reality. We can see the world around us, be with friends, on public transport or in front of a TV, and from the outside, look fine. Internally, however, it can feel like we are viewing the world from behind a thick screen we can't get through, unable to interact with it. We can feel desperately alone.
- **Defensive.** When shame is the feeling of being bad, it can make us feel that everyone around us can see all the ways in which we are bad in that moment. Survivors can feel people around us scrutinising us. This doesn't have to be true for survivors to feel defensive.
- **Distrust.** Shame can make survivors doubt all relationships and even feel like we cannot trust the people in our lives.
- **Worthless.** Survivors often feel worthless when shame is activated. This can feel like extreme impostor syndrome or a sense that we are pathetic and lack value.
- **Depression.** Shame can feel like it is pulling us down into a depression. This can feel immovable and heavy.

Bodily

- **Hot.** Some survivors can feel our bodies getting hot and even physically sweating when shamed. We get red in the face, feeling our cheeks warm up.
- **Heavy eyes.** Some survivors can become sleepy, even in charged situations like an argument with a family member or loved one. During confrontation or in

shaming situations, we may start to feel our eyes getting heavy, yawn, and need to sleep. The shame gets too much, and the body starts to shut down.

- **Shrinking.** Many survivors, when shamed, try to make our bodies as small as possible. We can become sunken, hunching our shoulders, wrapping our arms across our chest, or wanting to curl into a ball.
- **Excess energy in the body.** Some survivors can feel parts of our bodies shake, like hands or restless feet. Others might experience physical tics, like blinking, twitching, or nerves pulsing in the eyelids. Still others may experience sickness in the stomach or a tightness across the chest. This can even lead to panic attacks.
- **Digestion.** Shame, as well as stress, can affect our body's appetite. Some survivors may reach for food to comfort ourselves while others may experience a physiological response that restricts digestion and causes stomach aches.

Behavioural

- **Conscious dissociation.** Some survivors deliberately numb a shame response by using cigarettes, alcohol, or drugs. This can also feel like a freeze or flight response. I refer to it as *conscious dissociation* because some survivors won't dissociate unconsciously. Instead, we deliberately alter our consciousness with chemicals to avoid or pacify the shame.
- **Explode outward.** Some people need to throw our shame as far away from us as possible, like a live grenade. Some survivors use the term *shame-rage* to describe the change in our behaviour when shame is paired with an emotional reaction like anger. For example, survivors might try to control anger but become bad-tempered or snappy with loved ones. Some survivors can bottle anger up for a period, leading to a delayed explosion. Other survivors can feel the need to harm ourselves using self-harm or risky behaviours, and others may take our aggression out on something, for example, hitting walls, slamming doors, etc.
- **Become submissive.** Shame can rob a survivor of any agency when speaking to another person. We can say, 'I don't know what I want', or 'Do whatever you want to do'. This passive attitude to decision making can be difficult in social situations, as when a couple has an argument. It is, however, self-protective. It is the mind of the survivor playing dumb or going limp (much like the flop response; see page 28). Survivors may be in an argument with our partner or a stressful situation at work and suddenly find ourselves completely submissive. Here, our mind is powering down, and we become compliant to the needs or demands of the other person.
- **Become selfish.** Shame can make survivors feel like we are the centre of the universe. The acute feeling of shame can make us appear selfish, not considering other people's emotions or feelings. The truth is, shame can be so strong that there is no emotional room left for anyone else. This can make it difficult for

survivors who feel ashamed to judge our behaviours rationally or act in the way we might normally.

Reflective activity

With the three ways of breaking down shame: situation, automatic thoughts, and reactions in mind. Can you think of a recent situation where you felt shamed? Start small, before tackling something like abuse. Are you able to break down the situation, your thoughts and three reactions?

If you find yourself lost for words, you can borrow some of the reactions from the previous pages or use the Emotions Wheel on page 256. Below is an example of how someone may think about this, can you replace the example with your own situation?

Situation. Arrive at work on time, boss asks for a word later.

Automatic thoughts. What have I done wrong? Why is it always me?

Reactions:

1. **Emotion.** Nervous, irritated, confused.
2. **Bodily.** Knot in stomach, face starts to feel hot.
3. **Behavioural.** Scroll through social media, make a list of what could be wrong, skip lunch, snap at co-worker.

Because I have worked with survivors of all genders for a long time, I have noticed some additional reactions when survivors are exposed to shame over a significant period of time. These are not necessarily instant reactions to feeling shamed but are sustained ways of being or thinking that could originate from shame.

Intrusive thoughts. Survivors can get trapped in a repeated cycle of shameful thoughts about themselves for a long time. They constantly focus on the things they think are wrong about themselves and become highly critical. This can become habitual, automatic behaviour. A survivor can think something negative about themselves every moment of the day. Some experience this as repetitive or intrusive thinking. This can be mistaken as a form of obsessive compulsive disorder (OCD) when unwanted thoughts start to take over, though it can actually be symptomatic of complex post-traumatic stress disorder (cPTSD).

The two P's. Shame may affect our relationship with work or tasks. For some survivors, this manifests in a form of *perfectionism*. Driven by shame, they cannot allow anything in life to be less than perfect, rehearsing conversations in their heads and feeling sick at the thought of getting something wrong. Conversely, in other survivors, shame manifests as *procrastination*, leaving them unable to start anything, despite knowing how to. They might feel sleepy, distracted, anxious, or do anything else to avoid starting what they need to complete.

Avoidant behaviour. This behaviour can be subtle and hard to spot. It occurs when a survivor changes their behaviour to avoid being noticed. For example, they might not say anything in a work meeting or take themselves out of situations where they feel they may be shamed, like socialising with friends.

The theories of shame

Whether you are a survivor or an ally, understanding how shame has been viewed in psychology can help us to understand how it can affect us in our own lives. It can also help us to avoid some of the stigma about sexual abuse that psychology has helped to perpetuate in the past.

Historically, different therapists promote different ideas about shame and where it comes from. Some believe shame is just a painful emotion that is individual to each person, requiring that therapists work to understand what it means for each of their clients individually. Others believe that shame is a form of defence against something too painful to acknowledge. These different beliefs are born out of the psychoanalytic tradition, which has been around since the early 1890s and was established by Austrian neurologist Sigmund Freud, who is largely thought of as the 'father of modern psychology'.

One theory Freud argued was that shame functions as a defence mechanism against something that feels forbidden or dangerous. For Freud, this almost always led back to sex or early parental experiences. He might say shame is a reaction against a desire that is too dangerous to admit: 'A person may be led to feel shame or embarrassment, which is only a reaction against the excitement and, in a roundabout way, is an admission of it'.[1]

Having worked with sexual abuse survivors for a long time, I do not believe that shame is a defence against a buried feeling of excitement toward the abuse. I use Freud's quote here only because a great many survivors have been harmed by mental health professionals who reinforce this belief. Countless times, I have heard stories from survivors about a doctor or therapist who told them they needed to admit that a part of them enjoyed the abuse before they could heal. This is deeply unethical, damaging, and untrue.

Some survivors may find this myth about shame complicated because they have mixed feelings about their perpetrator. They may have been shown 'kindness' from the perpetrator in a time where they had little or no kindness. This is common in childhood abuse or where grooming occurs. Experiencing these feelings can make feelings of shame even worse. We will look at this further later on in the chapter.

If shame is not a defence, like this Freud quote suggests, where does it come from? Psychologists have done work around what are called *basic emotions*. This research suggests that all human beings have a limited number of biologically and psychologically basic emotions. In the 1970s, Paul Ekman worked to identify universal emotions, theorising that some basic human emotions (happiness/enjoyment, sadness, anger, fear, surprise, disgust, and contempt) are innate and shared by everyone.[2] Other studies suggest different numbers of basic emotions, from five to 27! (If you want a good example of this theory of emotions, watch Pixar's film *Inside Out* (2015), the story of five universal emotions – Fear, Anger, Joy, Disgust, and Sadness – inside an 11-year-old girl's head as she goes through the process of moving to a new city).

Many studies that attempt to summarise basic emotions fail to talk about or recognise shame. This is perhaps because shame is a socially learned emotion. Antonio Damasio, a neurobiologist and professor of psychology, philosophy, and neurology at the University of Southern California, theorises that we develop secondary emotions later in our early life development, probably around the same time we develop a sense of self (Damasio, 1999).[3] Shame is an example of one of these secondary emotions. Newborn babies are not born with shame, but by the time they are two years old, they have learned it. Children learn shame over time by coming into contact with the people around them, including parents or carers. A 2010 literature review of shame studies conducted by Matos and Pinto-Gouveia set out to explore the premise that shame has similar properties to traumatic memories, intrusive thoughts, flashbacks, and dissociation. Shame-proneness seems to have trauma-like origins in early negative rearing experiences, namely experiences of shaming, abandonment, rejection, emotional negligence or emotional control, and several forms of abusive, critical and/or harsh parental styles.

They tell us that '[s]hame-proneness seems to have trauma-like origins in negative rearing experiences, namely negligence, or emotional control, and several forms of abusive, critical, and/or harsh parenting styles'.[4]

This quote feels especially powerful to me. It tells us shame can feel as powerful as trauma. Mix shame with the experience of sexual abuse, along with the stigma that survivors can experience and individual factors, such as disability, age, sexuality, or sexual preferences like BDSM, and we start to see how trauma and shame can build up and become completely debilitating.

5.2   Society and shame

It would be difficult to discuss shame without discussing its place in society. I don't think anyone escapes being shamed, either by a caregiver or the culture they are born into. Shame is a tool for maintaining the social order, and in this sense, it is necessary. Shame keeps people obeying the social norms that enable societies to exist. As children grow up, they are exposed to shame from the outside world, parents, and caregivers. Most parents don't mean to do this; however, the shame serves a useful function. I once heard a parent say to their child in a supermarket, 'Can you do up your shoelaces? I know you can; only babies need someone to do their laces for them'.

This comment may have shamed that child, but hopefully not too much. While I don't recommend trying to influence a child's behaviour through shame, I would *hope* moments like this serve to build up the child's tolerance for shame. Small and safe enough amounts of shame inoculate children against future shameful moments that are more psychologically harmful.

However, children who are often on the receiving end of shame can become negatively affected by it, particularly when language is used to exercise control over that child. Teachers, parents, and carers can use shame and shame-laced language and tone to control children in ways that don't inoculate and build up resistance to shame, but compound and worsen it. As Susan Miller, concludes in her monograph *The Shame Experience*,

> Parents teach their children the meaning of the words 'shame' and 'guilt' in part by tone of voice. Often 'shame' is used in context of the chastising injunction, 'You should be ashamed of yourself'. Perhaps even more effective is the interrogative, 'Aren't you ashamed of yourself?'[5]

Miller goes on to suggest that using shame in this way internalises it. The parent's implied tone communicates that the fault is within the child and invites punishment; however, the parent does not enact the punishment. The parent doesn't need to answer the question 'Aren't you ashamed of yourself?' because the child will do that for them, internally answering, 'Yes, I am bad'. The fault is planted inside the child, leaving them to punish themselves. The child now has all the tools they need to punish and shame themselves, even without anyone else present. Whenever they are socially awkward, fail exams, or are bad at sport, they can punish themselves: *Why am I so bad? Why are my classmates so much better than me?* They can also threaten themselves with shame: *I better get a good grade. I don't want to be a loser all my life!* The child can develop shame-prone thinking that stays with them into adult life.

Naturally, we do not want children or adults to go through life shaming themselves. However, undoing this shame-prone thinking requires self-reflection. Self-reflection is essential for changing how we think and feel. To self-reflect is to imagine a different way of being in the world. For example, it might be okay to not be good at sport or to fail an exam, but shame can become so enmeshed in a person's psyche that it blocks their ability to imagine any other way of being. It stops the essential self-reflection needed for long-term psychological change.

People who experience verbal shaming from a parent or caregiver in childhood often report other behaviours from the parent or caregiver that amplify shame:

- Lack of positive reinforcement or recognition of positive behaviour
- Absence of appropriate boundaries and discipline
- Neglect or absence of meeting emotional needs

- The use of 'conditions of worth' to influence behaviour (eg, *I will love you only if you tidy your room/do well at school/perform in a way that I want you to*)
- Public humiliation or punishment

A child who experiences some of these from a parent or caregiver will often find appropriate discipline from a teacher or youth worker extremely difficult. As a result, even the best ways of disciplining a shame-prone child can cause a shame response for that child. This can lead to anything from punishing self-thoughts or self-harm, sabotaging work or exams, or acts of aggression.

Shaming behaviour doesn't just come from parents. Shame can exist within cultural groups and collective identities. We often see this in certain religious groups. In Catholicism, for example, the idea of original sin tells us that the very act of being born is all it takes to have sin within us, and it can only be removed through baptism and penance through confession. Another group that can be particularly shame-prone is the LGBTQIA+ community. Much of modern society seeks to control, squash, or deny homosexuality in many different ways. In Western Europe and America, for example, so-called 'conversion therapy' is used as a way of 'curing' a person's homosexuality. Parents who feel ashamed of their LGBTQIA+ child might attempt to remove that shame by subjecting the child to conversion therapy, thus passing parents' shame on to the child. Sally Munt describes this process in her article 'Gay shame in a geopolitical context':

> Gay conversion therapies, for example, remain popular; they perpetuate the idea of a 'gay cure' often in the name of religious conformity. Gay conversion therapy is often imposed upon children by homophobic parents, who cannot face the shame of a gay son, indeed a high proportion of such patients are teenagers. These abused, predominantly Christian young men think they are sick, diseased and broken because they are gay; in an Orwellian cruelty the therapy is often described as a 'reparative therapy'. One of its main pioneers, Joseph Nicolosi (2016), claimed that there is no such thing as homosexuality and that everyone has a natural, and universal, heterosexuality. In 'reparative therapy' models, a failed heterosexual trajectory is blamed on emotional injury, a fallacious psychotherapeutic model of healing.[6]

These forms of oppression can manifest in internalised homophobia or transphobia when an external fear of sexuality in a society or family becomes internalised by an LGBTQIA+ person. Often, collective traumas faced by a marginalised group can be used by broader society to shame its members. The AIDS crisis of the 1980s and 1990s was not only traumatic for the gay community, but also became a source of public shaming with reports of a 'gay plague' and the spread of misinformation and stigma. Black people living in the legacy of the African diaspora may find that exposure to racist sentiments exacerbates internalised shame around their identity. Amber J. Johnson's study 'Examining associations between racism, internalised shame, and self-esteem among African Americans' found that the frequency of past-year racist events significantly predicted internalised shame.[7]

Some find shame so painful that feeling it provokes acts of abuse and violence. *Honour abuse*, for example, is not a specific offence, but a term that captures multiple types of abuse motivated by shame or the 'dishonouring' of a person's family or community. If a person behaves in a way that breaks the social rules of a community, it can lead to physical assault, forced marriage, rape, or harassment. Often women are the primary victims of this type of abuse; however, gay and disabled men are often targeted too.

Shame is truly embedded within society. Even without living through the experience of sexual abuse, men's internal architecture – how they think, behave, or take care of their health – can be negatively impacted by shame. This is why it is essential to tackle men's shame when it comes to recovery from sexual abuse.

5.3   Sexual abuse and shame

As we have seen, shame is often a tool for control. Parents can use it to make children behave, society uses it to keep its members behaving in acceptable ways, and individuals often use it to punish themselves. Perpetrators of sexual abuse also use shame to silence victims and protect themselves. These perpetrators are protected by society when it believes shaming myths about male survivors rather than victims.

Each person has their own individual relationship with shame. This relationship can be informed by abuse as well as experiences outside of abuse. School, parents or carers, disabilities, gender dysphoria, race, economic status, and sexuality can all be sources of shame depending on each individual's circumstances. When I give lectures about abuse and shame, I find it useful to break experiences down into developmental stages:

- Childhood
- Adolescence
- Adulthood

It's likely you'll find crossover between these developmental stages. If you were abused in childhood, you might still find much of the following 'Shame and abuse in adulthood' section relatable to your experience, and vice versa. The same goes for adolescence. This is because, though I break these experiences down for clarity, we often do not experience shame in such a tidy way.

As with every topic in this book, please remember to take your time with this section. In the groups I run, the sessions on shame can catch people by surprise. They can be far more difficult than expected, often transporting survivors back to a difficult time in their lives. Take breaks, use the grounding exercises in this book, and make sure you are in a comfortable place when reading. There is no need to rush this. Give yourself time; these pages will be waiting for you when you are ready!

Shame and abuse in childhood

Often, children who are abused find themselves deeply confused by the experience. They are too young to have the appropriate language or understanding to describe the abuse. They literally do not comprehend the concept nor have the vocabulary to describe the disturbing experience of such abuse. They cannot make sense of the experience for themselves, and this makes it almost impossible to tell anyone else. Children *can* understand the feelings of wrongness, otherness, and fear that abuse causes. This becomes especially confusing if the perpetrator is someone responsible for the care of the child, such as a parent, carer, teacher, sports coach, etc. The perpetrator may also show the child affection that seems appropriate. It can add additional confusion when the perpetrator gives appropriate care to the abused child, only to follow it with abuse. The abuse can be part of a pattern of behaviour from the perpetrator or a one-off event.

I often work with survivors who tell me a carer, parent, or responsible adult abused them but was also kind and treated them well. Survivors can often feel like this person in their life was 50 per cent good and 50 per cent abusive. The truth, however, is that to be sometimes good and sometimes abusive is an entirely damaging experience – 100 per cent abusive. The confusion, fear, and unpredictability this inconsistent treatment creates can continue well into adulthood and be life-altering for the child and their future relationships.

Once the child has grown up, they can struggle to have clear memories of the abuse. This is because when the abuse was happening, they didn't understand it. Childhood memories can also be hard to access when they are shrouded in secrecy (see page 43 for more on memory). The survivor may also hold on to fond feelings for the perpetrator if they seemed to give appropriate care. Both the inability to remember clearly and having mixed feelings for a perpetrator are difficult experiences and can fuel shame, as well as protecting the perpetrator.

The fact that children cannot fully comprehend that an adult who is meant to look after them could harm them is an important aspect of shame in childhood abuse. The concept of an adult who wants to harm a child is existentially damaging to children. If the child cannot accept that the adult is responsible for the harm, they internalise their feeling of 'wrongness'. It is easier for a child to believe that they are wrong than to believe an adult meant to protect is wrong. The shame is planted within the child because they do not have the cognitive tools to put the blame on the perpetrator. The shame keeps growing within the child unchallenged.

In some cases, the perpetrator will use this shame to control the child. Much like our earlier shaming parent, perpetrators can use language to compound shame, saying things like,

- Don't tell anyone or you will get me in big trouble.
- Don't tell anyone or you will be in big trouble.
- You don't want anything bad to happen to me, do you?

- This is our secret. If you tell anyone, you will really upset me.
- Don't ruin our special relationship.
- You will upset everyone if you tell.
- You don't want to be bad, do you?

Other perpetrators don't say anything to the child at all. This creates shame in the absence of anything else and can be so confusing that the child is left only with the feeling of wrongness, unable to understand what has happened.

Children and teens who are targeted by perpetrators have often already experienced shame. Children who grow up to have LGBTQIA+ identities can report feeling different or marginalised from an early age. They have already begun being pushed out of society and shamed even before they come out or fully understand their sexuality or gender. One stigmatising myth about male survivors is that it is a 'gay man's' problem, or, that abuse 'turns' someone gay or trans. In truth, however, children who grow up to have LGBTQIA+ identities are more likely to be targeted because they are already outsiders. Children growing up below the poverty line or in a minority community have a similar experience of being marginalised. They often cannot access certain social groups or resources or are 'othered' for their identity. This makes them vulnerable to shame as well as to perpetrators.

Child-on-child abuse can be equality confusing. In addition to all the previously mentioned circumstances (lack of clear memories, feelings of wrongness or shame), further complications can also arise. Because both the victim and the perpetrator are children, this form of abuse can be ignored. Even survivors can tell themselves that the abuse was simply 'experimentation' that is common in children. Adults who are responsible for a child's welfare may overlook this type of sexual abuse for the same reason, writing it off as 'kids will be kids'. Some adults find the idea of child-on-child sexual abuse too difficult or complicated to manage, so they ignore it.

It is really important to think about the power dynamics that can exist between children. This applies in all environments: in the local area, in school or class, even within the family. Understanding this can help professionals spot vulnerable children and help survivors in adulthood identify whether their childhood experience was abusive. Power imbalances can occur due to age or status, disability or cognitive ability, social and economic status, gender or heritage. The perpetrating child's circumstances could be abusive, including early sexualisation due to exposure to pornography, experiencing sexual abuse themselves, or some other form of neglect or abuse. Some children who are abused repeat the behaviour towards other children. It is important to note that this is not predetermined. Experiencing abuse at any time in your life does not mean you will go on to abuse others. For those who do, the situation is complex, positioning a survivor as both victim and perpetrator. This can happen at any age and demonstrates how violence is perpetuated throughout generations and communities (for more on this, see transformative justice (TJ) pages 184 & 217).

If you feel confused about whether you experienced childhood abuse by another child or children, it may come down to how you feel about these experiences. All the memorable evidence might point to experimentation, but you might feel like it was wrong or shameful. This likely points to some type of power imbalance, therefore qualifying it as potential abuse. This can be hard to come to terms with, but no one has the right to tell you what you did or didn't experience. Trusting how you feel and working to understand it can be crucial to understanding your experience of child-on-child sexual abuse.

Shame and abuse in adolescence

Modern Western societies often have a preoccupation with teenagers and their sexuality. Films, particularly horror films, are a good example. They often punish teenage characters for being sexuality active by killing them off early in the story. At the same time, however, they allow audiences to view enough of the promiscuous behaviour to be secretly excited by it. Within the first four minutes of Steven Spielberg's film *Jaws* (1975), we are introduced to Chrissie Watkins. She sits on a beach at night, but when she sees a boy she likes, she invites him into the ocean. We see her strip naked and dive into the waves, kicking her legs up in the air seductively, only to be attacked and killed by the man-eating shark. This cinematic trope appears in the real world when assumptions are made about teenagers' sexuality. Society says that teenagers have no respect or responsibility, are always 'horny', and should have their sexuality policed while simultaneously sexualising them in film, music, and social media. Often the only voice left out of the discussion about teenagers' sexuality is that of teenagers themselves.

Society's double standards about teenagers either sexualise them or punish them for being sexual. Because of this, teenagers who experience sexual abuse are often dismissed, blamed and undermined. The following lists include some examples of what society says about teenagers who have been abused.

Sexualising statements about teenage survivors

- They knew what they were doing.
- They seduced the perpetrator.
- Kids these days are always thinking about sex.
- He was just being a typical horny boy.
- He should consider himself lucky.
- They are old enough to consent; it can't be abuse.

Judgemental and punishing statements about teenage survivors

- They deserve to be raped if they act like a slut.
- If they don't want to be assaulted, they shouldn't dress like that.
- He was leading them on; what did he expect was going to happen?

- They are playing the victim/want attention.
- If you're going to get out-of-control drunk, what do you expect to happen?

In society's eyes, teenagers either know what they are doing and want and are ready for sexual attention (it's common for perpetrators in court to describe teenage survivors as 'mature for their age' as a way to justify abuse), or they bring on the abuse by behaving in certain 'shameful' ways. This attitude assumes teenagers are developmentally mature and not emotionally vulnerable. Teenagers appear mature for lots of reasons. Some who have faced challenges in early life appear mature or take on adult responsibilities, such as caring for younger children. Other teenagers who find themselves at odds with society – such as neurodivergent, disabled, or LGBTQIA+ young people – can seem more mature because they must navigate a society that is not set up for them. Black children and teenagers are particularly vulnerable to being sexualised and having people assume they are more mature that they are. This issue falls under the broader problem of 'adultification'. According to Davis and Marsh,

> adultification is when notions of innocence and vulnerability are not afforded to certain children. This is determined by people and institutions who hold power over them. When adultification occurs outside of the home it is always founded within discrimination and bias.
>
> There are various definitions of adultification, all relate to a child's personal characteristics, socio-economic influences and/or lived experiences. Regardless of the context in which adultification takes place, the impact results in children's rights being either diminished or not upheld.[8]

Adultification perpetuates ideas that not only sexualise and punish teenagers but also lead to institutional abuse. In 2022, members of the Metropolitan Police in London sexually assaulted a 15-year-old Black girl in her school in Hackney by strip-searching her without another adult present while she was on her period on the suspicion she was carrying cannabis. This girl, known as Child Q later said,

> Someone walked into the school, where I was supposed to feel safe, took me away from the people who were supposed to protect me and stripped me naked, while on my period.
>
> On the top of preparing for the most important exams of my life. I can't go a single day without wanting to scream, shout, cry or just give up.
>
> I feel like I'm locked in a box, and no one can see or cares that I just want to go back to feeling safe again, my box is collapsing around me, and no one wants to help.[9]

It is important for all teenagers to try out acting grown-up. This is part of becoming more independent and separating from their families. They feel mature and independent, like they are in control, making their own decisions. This is an important part of developing into an adult. Observers of this behaviour may overestimate such young people's maturity, missing their emotional vulnerability, which is far more childlike. This creates an environment in which perpetrators can assume teenagers' sexual maturity, ignoring their emotional vulnerability, and society can judge adolescent victims harshly, compounding the trauma of abuse.

This leaves teenagers trapped. Some may experience abuse but feel like they are allowing it to happen or consenting to it. Because of their childlike need for love and approval, they may even seek out the affections of their abuser with a perceived sense of being grown-up when, in truth, they are extremely vulnerable. This can occur in the home or through dating or hookup apps, social media, or seeking out spaces where anonymous sex happens. This can make the abuse extremely difficult to come to terms with later. Survivors may internalise all society's judgements about teenagers, judge their own behaviour through this lens, and thus, invite the shame to engulf them, rather than blaming the perpetrator.

The truth is, teenagers are growing and developing at an extraordinary rate. At no other time in a person's life (with the exception of toddlerhood), do they change physically, hormonally, and mentally as quickly as they do in adolescence. Because of this, teenagers are living paradoxes. They need the love, support, and attention of safe adults, peers, and community leaders, while needing to feel independent and adult at the same time. This leaves them vulnerable to those who exploit this paradox to target teenagers for many types of abuse, from sexual abuse to political or religious extremism to gang involvement. When abuse happens, teenagers are quick to blame and shame themselves. Sadly, society is also quick to blame them. All of this protects perpetrators and keeps teenagers imprisoned by shame and abuse.

Shame and abuse in adulthood

In 2023, I recorded the second series of my podcast, The Trauma Talks. Each episode investigated challenges and coping strategies associated with experiencing a different type of trauma. We looked at many different experiences, from birth PTSD (PTSD originating from the process of giving birth or medical mistreatment during labour) to prisons, and of course, sexual abuse. The episode about male survivors of sexual abuse in adulthood had two guests who were experts through lived experience. When one of them, Steve, was asked what stops men from getting help after abuse, he said,

> Shame means I can't tell anybody; I can't tell anybody this. In the case of my shame, I did tell a rape group, and they said it doesn't happen to men – shame internalised! This was back in 2000, but it was shame upon shame upon shame. I was wrong, which is the definition of shame; there was something wrong with me.[10]

Steve's story is not unique. In the vast majority of recovery groups I've run, at least one group member has had someone tell them sexual abuse doesn't happen to men. When society tells male survivors that one of the most painful experiences in their lives can't happen, it leaves men with deep shame and isolation. No wonder it can take decades for men to disclose, if they do so at all.

When we do see examples of male sexual abuse in adulthood, it is often trivialised or used for humour. Male survivors often can't win. Their trauma is either denied or used as a punchline. Here are two films that use different types of sexual abuse for humour.

No Hard Feelings (2023)

In this 2023 comedy, Jennifer Lawrence plays a 32-year-old woman, Maddie, who needs money to pay her housing tax. She sees an advert in an online directory from parents secretly trying to set up their 19-year-old son, Percy, with an older woman to coerce him into losing his virginity before university. For this, Maddie will be given a car. Throughout the film we see Maddie

- Constantly making sexual advances, even when asked not to (at one point, Percy uses Mace spray because he feels so threatened)
- Using alcohol to lower underage Percy's inhibitions, then rubbing herself on his lap, making him visibly uncomfortable
- Attempting to isolate Percy from his friends by being rude to them and preventing him from attending a house party with peers his own age
- Aggressively shouting at him, forcing him to strip naked and skinny dip with her
- Attempting to befriend him, making it easier to coerce him into sex

The film plays all of this for laughs, but when we compare Maddie's actions to multiple grooming models, we see plenty of crossover:

- Gain access to a victim and build trust with them and their family
- Isolate the victim from peers and support network
- Use substances to lower inhibitions or remove capacity for consent
- Desensitise the victim to sexual contact
- Maintain control over the victim

YouTube comments for the trailer are largely positive:

- I just saw this movie, it's one of the best I've seen in years.
- The 'kidnapping' scene got me rolling on the floor screaming.
- I watched it with my mom and during this scene we cried from laughter. Great movie.[11]

Generally, I avoid comparing male and female experiences of sexual abuse, as it can become unnecessarily divisive. However, the double standard in this film feels stark. It's hard to image a comedy made in 2023 in which a 32-year-old man is hired to coerce sex from a 19-year-old girl. It's also notable, that while the 19-year-old boy is arguably a victim in this film, his parents also exploit Maddie's economic and housing instability, coercing her into a sexual relationship she may not have freely consented to.

Get Hard (2015)

Get Hard is a film released in 2015 about a white man, James King, played by Will Ferrell. When James is sentenced to prison, he asks the one Black man he knows, Darnell, played by Kevin Hart, to prepare him. James's main motivation is fear of prison rape, and it becomes the film's entire narrative. Within this narrative, the film uses racial caricatures and homophobia to ultimately repeat the same 'James is scared of rape' joke in different situations.

As with *No Hard Feelings*, we see many positive comments on *Get Hard*'s YouTube trailer:

- This was a great film!! 10/10 hilarious, well-acted and captivating.
- I laughed to the point of hysterical hoarseness the ENTIRE running time!!
- A comedic A+ for me.[12]

I'm not making a judgement on whether these films are good or not. I'm not a film critic. However, they are both good illustrations of how society can easily laugh at grooming and rape when the violence is directed towards men. These films are an expression of society's attitudes towards male survivors, steeped in toxic masculinity (for more on toxic masculinity, see page 69). It is no wonder men feel shame about their experience and do not risk coming forward to disclose abuse. When films belittle experiences of sexual violence, survivors may belittle their own experience in the same way, not seeing anywhere in society where their experience is taken seriously.

Society doesn't just shame men about sexual abuse itself, but also the circumstances around the abuse. If an adult man is abused in a men's sauna or at a sex party, he may be shamed for acting promiscuously or for his sexuality. If a man is abused by a woman, he may be viewed as lucky or weak. If a man freezes during an attack, he may be told he should have fought, and if an older man is assaulted then he may be told he should be grateful for the attention.

Many aspects of adult male abuse that are considered shameful, fuelled by society's attitudes towards men and adult survivors. Following are of some of them.

Shame about trauma response

The vast majority of people freeze when abused, regardless of gender, age, physical ability or disability, or identity. Freezing is often the response that our body and mind consider safest because it can minimise the physical damage of an assault and prevent the attack from escalating. On most occasions, our mind and body decide that freezing is the trauma response most likely to lead to survival (see page 28 for more on trauma responses). However, society also considers freezing to be shameful and unmasculine. 'Why didn't you fight back?' is a refrain men often hear from loved ones and professionals. I've even heard accounts of therapists saying to their clients, 'A part of you must have wanted it, or you would have fought them off'.

This type of shame is particularly powerful inside survivors' own heads. Often, we find ourselves wondering why we behaved like we did during abuse. Even if we know all about trauma responses and how the brain works, a part of us still shames ourselves for not fighting or running. This can create an internal conflict where survivors hear two voices in our head: one understands how common freezing is, that it was the normal thing to do and may have helped us survive, while the other voice blames and shames us for freezing and not fighting abusers off. This argument can go on for years in survivors' heads after an abuse.

Shame about the perpetrator

Men face all sorts of judgement based on the identity of our abuser. Being a victim of sexual abuse is in itself a violation of society's concept of masculinity, and this judgement only becomes harsher depending on the abuser's identity. Women are thought of as the 'weaker' sex and less physically strong. Being victimised by a woman can be especially shame-provoking for men. Our experience may be ignored or fetishised. For example, a woman putting a man in a situation where he is forced to have sex with her has become an erotic archetype in cinema and pornography.

Adult men abused by a wife or girlfriend may be accused of being 'under the thumb' or 'henpecked' by our abuser, rather than cohesively controlled and abused. A man in a same-sex couple may also find his abusive relationship dismissed as 'passionate', rather than being recognised for what it is: controlling and sexually abusive. Disabled men may depend on our perpetrator, leaving us trapped, relying on our abuser for essential care while also vulnerable to assault. Adult men from certain countries can be victims of forced marriage. While women are the most common victims of forced marriage, men make up 63 per cent and 55 per cent, respectively, of forced marriage victims who either are gay or have diminished mental capacity.[13]

Whatever the circumstances, society has a hard time acknowledging certain types of perpetrators. Whether the perpetrator is a female or a partner, society makes judgements and applies a hierarchy of harm that says some perpetrators aren't as harmful as others. These judgements can imprison male survivors and keep them in relationships with their perpetrators for a long time, increasing the danger they are in and exacerbating feelings of shame.

Shame and victim blaming

Victim blaming occurs when an individual or social group, such as the media, social services, education providers, criminal justice professionals, or healthcare providers put some amount of responsibility on the survivor, either partial or complete. Victim blaming is an act of shaming a survivor, using our identity or behaviour to belittle and degrade us. If a rape case goes to court, it is common for the legal team defending the perpetrator to verbally attack the survivor, bringing into question their motives or behaviour. Many segments of society, both in the criminal justice system and the news and social media, judge and shame survivors for the circumstances around the abuse.

Victim blaming is common in our society, and survivors of all genders and identities experience it. LGBTQIA+ men who attend chemsex parties or saunas, for example, often have their experiences diminished and are shamed. Straight society is quick to judge LGBTQIA+ men and their sex lives. Within chemsex culture some men shame those who experience sexual abuse. Some survivors of assault during chemsex find that other gay men belittle the rape, saying it is part and parcel of the culture and survivors should 'get over it'. This experience can not only be shaming but can fuel internalised homophobia and self-loathing among LGBTQIA+ men.

Some straight men may experience this shame differently. They may never disclose an abuse because they do not want people to assume they are gay or doing something they shouldn't. The way society judges LGBTQIA+ men also holds straight men prisoner, preventing them from seeking support for fear of persecution and shame.

The truth is, where you were, what decisions you made and any other circumstances around the abuse don't matter. Ultimately, abuse comes down to a person or people using power over another to disregard, discount, or ignore their right to consent.

Shame and identity

Survivors with different identities must fight various barriers when seeking support after sexual abuse. This is particularly true of survivors from underrepresented communities. For example, Black men may find it particularly shaming to deal with sexual abuse. In some Black communities, the social norm is to 'just get on with it' without seeking support. This means that sexual abuse never gets talked about and survivors are never able to process their pain and trauma. Even if a Black survivor does seek support, a shortage of Black therapists and healthcare professionals means Black survivors may struggle to find a service or reparative experience where they feel understood. It is also common for trans men to not tell healthcare professionals about past trauma for fear that their hormones or treatment will be stopped. Many trans people have told me about doctors who withhold hormones assuming that trans identity is the result of abuse. Trans people may also internalise the idea that abuse caused their trans identity. This compounds the shame around their gender and identity. Rather than being able to see themselves as complex and nuanced human beings, they may view their own identity through the lens of sexual abuse.

Abuse and assumptions

Disabled men are too often overlooked in all parts of society. Both men with visible and nonvisible disabilities face non-disabled people belittling their experience. Non-disabled people often make assumptions about disabled bodies or minds and their attractiveness. This leads to disabled men hearing, 'Who would want to have sex with you?' This kind of comment is damaging and wrong on many levels. It misunderstands the nature of sexual abuse, assuming such abuse is about attraction rather than power. Simultaneously, it removes disabled men's right to relationships, sex, or intimacy.

These attitudes mean disabled men who report abuse are less likely to be taken seriously. On top of this, it is often much harder for disabled men to report because they can face access difficulties. For example, someone who is d/Deaf or deaf-blind/DeafBlind may not be able to access communication tools to report abuse. Abusers may take away or monitor technology use. Disabled people also may not have adequate economic means to acquire such devices. All of these barriers can feel like a clear message to disabled men that their experience or trauma is less important. Similar to other groups, disabled men can internalise these ideas and shame themselves.

There are many ways adult male survivors can feel shamed. This is because shame is a relational emotion. As we have seen, babies are not born with shame but learn it from those around them. This is related to their relationship with the environment they are born into. Adult male survivors are in a relationship with a society that constantly judges and shames us over who the perpetrator was and how we responded to the trauma, as well as making assumptions about our identity or behaviour. This relationship makes it difficult for men to break free of shame; in fact, it does the opposite. It keeps men living in constant shame, which creates feelings and behaviours that harm men and those around us.

This chapter is a bit of a monster. Not only is it long, but it is dense. We looked at a survivor's testimony (thank you again TDM) and broke down shame using some CBT. We've looked at some theories on shame and how it operates in society. We've also explored how sexual abuse can both plant the seed of shame and act as a catalysis for shame around identity.

What I haven't done is offer a clear-cut definition of what shame is. This is because shame is multifaceted. According to the CBT model, shame involves an individual's set of beliefs about themselves, their bodily reactions and their behaviours. To try and summarise shame as any one thing that can be applied to everyone – all experiences, identities, beliefs – feels too big.

What I will say, though, is that shame is powerful – maybe the most powerful emotion humans feel. While writing this chapter, I have had nightmares, disproportionately big emotional reactions to friends or colleagues, poor sleep, and bodily memories that resurface from the past. As in a séance, I have conjured up my own shame from the deep, simply by objectively writing about it. My colleague

Katherine Cox describes shame as a 'vampire emotion', thriving in the dark, feeding on us when we are alone, sapping our life when the lights are out. However, when it's exposed to the light, shame can be destroyed. In this case, the 'light' is connection with people and communities who make us feel understood, believed, and loved. It is connection that provides an antidote to the silencing and disturbing experience of shame. For some, this connection starts with therapy or a support group. For those who don't feel ready to start talking about abuse and shame directly, simple interactions such as participating in sport groups, meeting up for tea, walking, or gardening can help. Even an online group accessed via chatrooms or social media can help to promote connection and start to take the sharp edges off shame.

I haven't come across any quick fixes for shame, but I have seen people consciously shine a light on what they find shameful. By shining that light, they allow other people to see some of their shame, and, amazingly, it does start to feel a little easier. For some of you, reading this book may be that first step. If it is, I think that is remarkable. Shame often doesn't allow us to take in compliments, so I'm going to repeat that: I think you are remarkable.

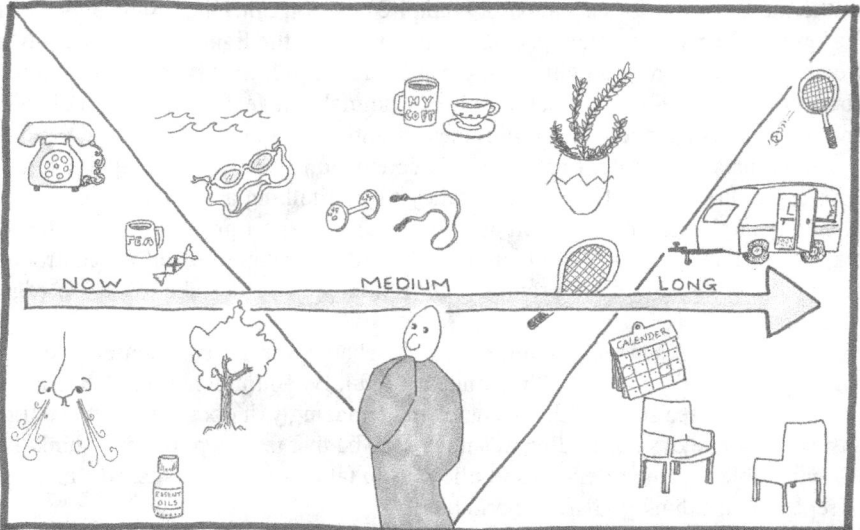

Now, Medium, & Long

It can help to categorise the strategies that help you cope with anxiety, stress, or cPTSD symptoms into things you can do now, things you can plan to do in the medium term, and things that can help in the long term.

By doing this, we not only have strategies to hand that help us immediately, but we can work helpful things into our weeks and months that contribute to our ability to cope long term.

These are just suggestions, they won't work or be appropriate for everyone. On a blank page in this book, why not write down a few ideas that fit into these 3 categories of things that help you cope now, in the medium term, and long term

NOW...	MEDIUM...	LONG...
Call a friend to chat	Plan an activity in your week (like swimming)	Book a short break or promise yourself a quiet weekend where you relax and do nice things for yourself
Make a tea or have a strong flavoured sweet	Arrange to have tea or coffee with a friend	
Use breathing exercises	Plan a time to do physical activity - anything from the gym to visiting a nice outdoor space	Stay committed to your new hobby
Change your environment, like visiting a local park or taking yourself into a different room.		Find a therapist who works for you
Find a smell that you enjoy - this could be an essential oil, hand cream, or scented candle	Try and find a new hobby, for example, tennis, craft workshops, online support groups	Book nice things in your calendar, for example, look up free things to do in your area, a cinema trip, gym classes, time with friends
	Buy yourself a 'hard to kill' pot plant and look after it	

www.jeremysachs.com   @JeremySachs_

For A4 and printable versions of this worksheet, visit www.jeremysachs.com

For A4 and printable versions of this worksheet, visit www.jeremysachs.com

Resources

Anxiety Is Really Strange *by Steve Haines*

ISBN: 9781848193895

This is an illustrated comic book that goes into detail about anxiety and our brains.

Baby Reindeer (2024)

This Netflix series, developed by Richard Gadd, explores several themes of abuse and power, including stalking and sexual violence. Themes of shame, abusive relationships, and power.

Signposting

CALM

www.thecalmzone.net

This organisation is a services and campaigning suicide prevention charity that provides support to all genders.

Notes

1 Sigmund Freud, *Jokes and Their Relation to the Unconscious*, ed. J. Strachey (London: Hogarth Press, 1960).
2 Paul Ekman, 'Universal emotions', Paul Ekman Group, 2024. www.paulekman.com/universal-emotions, accessed 3 June 2024.
3 Antonio Damasio, *The Feeling of What Happens* (Orlando, FL: Harcourt, 2010).
4 Marcela Matos and José Pinto-Gouveia, 'Shame as a traumatic memory', *Clinical Psychology and Psychotherapy* 17, no. 4 (Jul–Aug 2010): 299–312, 6.
5 Susan Miller, *The Shame Experience* (Hillsdale, NJ: Analytic Press, 1985), 170.
6 Sally R. Munt, 'Gay shame in a geopolitical context', *Cultural Studies* 33, no. 2 (7 February 2018): 223–248, 9, https://doi.org/10.1080/09502386.2018.1430840, accessed 2 August 2024.
7 Amber J. Johnson, Examining associations between racism, internalized shame, and self-esteem among African Americans, *Cogent Psychology* 7, no. 1 (2020): 6, doi: 10.1080/23311908.2020.1757857.
8 Jahnine Davis and Nicholas Marsh, 'Boys to men: The cost of "adultification" in safeguarding responses to Black boys', *Critical and Radical Social Work* 8, no. 2 (2020): 255–259.
9 Jim Gamble and Rory McCallum, *Local Child Safeguarding Practice Review: Child Q* (London: City of London & Hackney Safeguarding Children Partnership, March 2022). https://chscp.org.uk/wp-content/uploads/2022/03/Child-Q-PUBLISHED-14-March-22.pdf, accessed 2 August 2024.
10 'Male Survivors of Sexual Abuse in Adulthood', *The Trauma Talks*, series 2, episode 1 (Apple Podcasts, 10 May 2023), https://podcasts.apple.com/gb/podcast/the-trauma-talks-podcast/id1517405491?i=1000612318642.

11 Sony Pictures Entertainment, '*No Hard Feelings*: Official Red Band Trailer', YouTube, www.youtube.com/watch?v=P15S6ND8kbQ&t=1s, accessed 18 July 2024.

12 Warner Bros. Pictures, '*Get Hard*', YouTube, www.youtube.com/watch?v=jTi-h6zN DLg, accessed 18 July 2024.

13 UK Foreign, Commonwealth and Development Office, 'Forced Marriage Unit statistics 2020', UK Home Office, 1 July 2021. www.gov.uk/government/statistics/forced-marri age-unit-statistics-2020/forced-marriage-unit-statistics-2020, accessed 2 August 2024.

Chapter 6

Relationships and family

Chapter Contents

My relationships and self-esteem

My parents weren't bad to me growing up. I always thought they did their best and I turned out okay. I didn't think they had anything to do with the relationships I would constantly end up in. These relationships were mostly loveless and eventually sexless. For years I would just say 'yes' to anyone who wanted to date me. I would get into relationships telling myself 'My attraction will grow', or when things were bad, 'the world doesn't owe me happiness or a good relationship, just settle'. Mostly, this meant that my relationships would last about two years, then fall apart. I'd need to move out and start again. I would feel bad, because I couldn't end any of these unhappy relationships. I'd rely on these poor women to become so miserable with me they would break up. I could have stayed in a bad relationship forever.

In my early thirties I ended up in a relationship with a woman who I knew was wrong for me, our first big fight came three months in when she accused me of being untrustworthy. She pushed me into a wardrobe door, breaking my little finger. Instead of leaving, I found myself apologising to her. I soon lost interest in sex, but she would instigate it, and I would be terrified to say I didn't want to. She would forcefully touch and grope me. I would freeze, fearful she'd get physical again. One time, I said I wanted to break up and the usual cycle happened, she would get physical, then force 'make up sex' and the next day nothing changed. I was trapped. This went on for three years.

Eventually I got out, she threatened me, as did her family. I had to leave all my belongings; I never got them back, but I was free.

DOI: 10.4324/9781003423331-6

Many years after, in therapy, I realised my parents never explicitly harmed me. But my mum drank, often being distant and unresponsive. My dad worked a lot and was angry and unapproachable. While I don't blame them entirely, they could never emotionally connect with me. I can see now how my lack of self-esteem started in childhood, with removed, scary, and disinterested parents, and how this could lead to the abusive relationship. It's hard to realise that parents who do their best, still might not be good enough.

Anonymous

Our relationships can hold up a mirror that reflects the impact of sexual abuse. Past abuse can infiltrate our present relationships, negatively affecting them. Historic sexual abuse can become conspicuous in arguments, first dates, children's birthday parties, disagreements, or positive interactions when we are in a relationship with another person. Abuse doesn't respect boundaries or allow us to compartmentalise, no matter how much we try. It can surface in every type of relationship because sexual abuse is a relational trauma that can damage all future relationships in a survivor's life.

We explore the complexity between abuse and relationships in every chapter of this book. In Chapter 2, we learn about our relationship to trauma responses and how those responses affect our everyday lives. Chapter 3, we look at the Drama Triangle and how survivors can get stuck in relationship patterns. We also examine ACEs, a model that looks at childhood relationships and their developmental impact. Chapter 4 explores our relationships with masculinity and the society we live in. Chapter 5 addresses relationships that have shamed us. Chapter 7 focuses on sexual relationships, and Chapter 8 on building trust with others. Chapter 9 discusses how to tell people about our abuse, Chapter 10 looks at our relationship with coping strategies, and Chapter 11 focuses on our relationship with our future. Chapter 12 is for allies of survivors and how they may better support their relationship with male survivors and themselves.

Sexual abuse often causes difficult patterns to form in relationships, and why wouldn't it? Abuse can be life-altering; of course the aftermath would impact us and those around us. Past trauma can trap us in toxic patterns with family or friends. Alternatively, we may find ourselves consistently dating people who are not good for us. We can feel stuck, like we must either submit to a life of inadequate relationships or constantly fight for people who don't deserve our energy. Being able to spot these patterns is a useful step towards breaking relationship habits that do not serve us.

6.1 Spotting relationship patterns

Survivors often find ourselves in challenging relationship patterns. These patterns can make healthy and well-meaning relationships feel unsafe; conversely, we may not notice negative patterns when we're in unsafe or manipulative relationships. These patterns can be hard to spot and break out of. Following are some things we may say to ourselves that might indicate we've fallen into relationship patterns we feel powerless to change.

- **I keep letting harmful people into my life.** Due to our past trauma, some of us may have difficulty recognising red flags or signs we're being taken advantage of. This makes it challenging to set healthy boundaries and avoid toxic behaviours in others.
- **I never feel good enough.** Abuse can deeply affect our self-esteem and self-worth, leading to a persistent inner voice that tells us we are inadequate or unworthy of relationships. Additionally, we may agree to things we do not want in relationships, simply because we don't respect our own boundaries.
- **I never know how to end bad relationships.** We can struggle to end relationships due to fear of confrontation or being alone, often trapping us in unhealthy dynamics.
- **I feel walked over or taken for granted all the time.** We might struggle with assertiveness due to the abuse, making it hard to set and enforce boundaries.
- **If I separate from my partner/friend/family, I'll never find anyone else, so I just stay with them.** Fear of abandonment or being alone can trap us in unhealthy relationships, causing us to stay in them much longer than we should.
- **I never feel able to let my walls down and share my feelings.** Trust issues are common among survivors, which can make emotional vulnerability difficult and prevent us forming meaningful connections. We can even find ourselves pushing away people we wish we could connect with.

It can feel like these sorts of relationships just happen to us, like we are at the whims of the universe with no power to change them. *It's not my fault if toxic people are attracted to me*, we might say to ourselves, or, *It's like I have 'walk all over me' written on my forehead.* Other survivors may throw everything we have at relationships, trying to make them work and being disappointed or becoming locked in conflict. We might make statements like

- **I give so much to my relationships and receive so little back.** Some of us may overextend ourselves in relationships, often due to low self-worth and a desire to be valued or to make it work. This leads to imbalanced dynamics in which we are unappreciated. We may also tolerate others who do little to show us care or express how much they value us. Often, survivors can experience a mix of both, overextending ourselves for people who give little in return.
- **I stay with toxic people because I hope I can help them change.** Many of us stay in unhealthy relationships with the belief that we can fix or save our partner, often at the expense of our own wellbeing.

- **My relationships are always explosive.** Past trauma can lead to heightened emotional sensitivity and reactivity. This means we can co-create relationships with others who have similar levels of sensitivity and reactivity, leading to volatility.
- **I'm told I can be too much or overly dramatic or demanding.** Often survivors express our needs and emotions intensely or frequently, which others can perceive as overly dramatic or demanding.
- **My exes think I'm controlling, difficult, or even abusive.** Survivors often struggle with trust and seek to manage our environments to feel safe. Our trauma can manifest in behaviours that others perceive as controlling or difficult or that seem disproportionate to onlookers who have not experienced abuse.
- **I always overshare my emotions and experiences as soon as I like someone.** Some survivors may overshare early in relationships as a way to quickly establish intimacy and trust, which can overwhelm the other person. As a result, survivors may regret oversharing or feel ashamed of ourselves for wanting to be honest and open.

Some survivors get completely stuck in a way of being, we might say,

- **I don't even know how to find a relationship.** Survivors may struggle to recognise what a healthy relationship looks like or where to begin in seeking one, often due to our past traumatic experiences or a lack of positive relationship role models.
- **I always settle for whoever shows an interest, regardless of whether I like them or not.** Low self-esteem or a fear of rejection can lead survivors to accept relationships with individuals who may not be compatible or respectful, compromising our own needs and desires.
- **I trauma bond with other survivors, and the relationship becomes solely about our trauma.** Shared traumatic experiences can create strong bonds between survivors, but if they are not managed carefully, these relationships may become centred around the trauma, hindering personal growth and healing.
- **I keep people who are bad for me around because if I don't, I won't have any friends/partners/family.** Fear of abandonment or isolation can lead survivors to maintain connections with toxic or harmful individuals, even when we recognise the negative impact on our wellbeing.

You might identify with one, two, or many of these patterns from any of the three categories, and that is to be expected. These patterns often represent our attempts to get our needs met and feel safe. On top of this, some groups of men may experience continuous relationship danger that is unique to specific identities. A trans man, for example, might not only have to manage his sexual trauma when he dates, but he might also have to navigate the violence confronting the trans community daily – especially in dating or sexual environments. A disabled man abused by a family member might also rely on the same family member for support, keeping him locked in a harmful relationship. A bisexual man previously abused by a man may never feel safe enough to come out, act on his sexual or romantic feelings towards men or be his authentic self in relationships because he believes men are inherently dangerous and abusive. In short, sexual abuse makes relationships challenging, and these challenges intersect with our identity, circumstance, how we view the world and how the world views us.

While we might not be able to make the whole world safe for survivors, we can start to interrogate some of the relationship patterns that bring us distress. This isn't easy. If we fear abandonment, struggle to trust, or feel shame, these feelings can hold us back. Often, this is where therapy can play a role; it is not possible to heal in isolation from the hurt caused in a relationship, the reparation needs to also be done in a relationship. It's also why it is important when you enter into therapy to find a therapist you feel a rapport with. Therapy can be a place where these feelings come up, and the therapeutic relationship should allow you the opportunity to practise sitting with them. Rapport facilitates sharing these feelings with your therapist and thinking together about what they mean and how they affect your life. This process can simultaneously calm our feelings of shame and abandonment while challenging us to examine the behaviour patterns that hold us back.

If you do recognise your patterns listed here, you might try highlighting them and starting to ask yourself which past experiences might have caused you to feel like this? What needs are you trying to meet? Do you feel anger, unsafe, or shame? Are you reminded of someone who wanted to make you feel small or control you? If you withhold your emotions, what might you be trying to protect? These are important questions to get to the bottom of. Use the emotions wheel on page 256, if you struggle to identify how you feel.

One theory that offers insight into our behavioural patterns and interactions with others is transactional analysis (TA). TA encompasses various models of understanding transactions between individuals. In Chapter 2, page 54, we explored the Drama Triangle, a component of TA. Another part of TA that survivors in my groups find useful when thinking about their relationships, including current relationships and relationships with perpetrators, is the concept of *ego states*. Ego states were developed by psychiatrist Eric Berne in the late 1950s. They attempt to explain the different ways people in our lives effect our emotions and behaviour. There are three ego states we can occupy: parent, adult, and child ego states. Let's delve into each of them:

- **Parent ego state.** In this state, we may unconsciously think, emotionally react, or behave similarly to our parents or parental figures. For instance, someone whose parent withdrew when stressed might repeat this behaviour in adult relationships. The parent ego state can be nurturing, providing security and permission, or critical, where nothing is ever good enough and criticism is defended as supportive or *just wanting what's best for you.*

- **Adult ego state.** Here, we are less emotionally driven and more objective, making decisions based on facts and our present environment. It can be helpful to think of this state as a neutral information processor, the state in which we function in everyday environments.
- **Child ego state.** This state reflects behaviours, emotions, and thoughts reminiscent of childhood. People in this state may struggle to receive criticism and exhibit childlike tantrums, while others may handle complaints boastfully. The child ego state can be free, spontaneous, and playful or adaptive and compliant to external expectations.

(P) **Parent Ego State:** nurturing, providing security and permission, or critical, where nothing is ever good enough

(A) **Adult Ego State:** less emotionally driven and more objective, making decisions based on facts and our present environment

(C) **Child Ego State:** can be free, spontaneous and playful or adaptive and compliant to external expectations

These ego states are activated by those around us and influence our emotional responses and behaviour towards those people. You might notice this in your own life. For example, imagine you have a friend who you care about but is constantly making decisions you think are bad. They make their own life more difficult and become entangled in drama. One day, you meet up for a coffee, and they begin to tell you about their latest predicament. This may provoke one of several ego states in you, and you may respond in one of these three ways, depending on the ego state that's been activated:

1. You might find yourself getting frustrated with the friend. As you talk to them about their drama, you might need to fight the temptation to grab them by the shoulders and shake them, saying, 'For goodness' sake, why can't

you just grow up?' Their behaviour has awakened a critical parent ego state in you.

2. Alternatively, you might be overcome with worry as your friend explains their drama. You might think to yourself, *Gosh I wish they took better care of themselves*, or, *If only I could solve these problems for them*. This would also be a parental ego state, but a nurturing, protective one.

3. You might also find yourself being sucked into the drama. You may enjoy and encourage your friend's bad decisions, really relishing the retelling of disastrous stories and things going wrong. This could be your free child ego state, uninhibited by worry or discipline.

A person could have many different responses to any given situation. Personally, I know that different environments and people can invoke several ego states within me. Whenever I get together with my best friend, we instantly become silly and playful, and my free child ego state comes out to play. If I find myself in academic settings, on the other hand, even as a guest lecturer, I can feel shame-prone and compliant, my adaptive child is provoked, I often have to remind myself I am, in fact, an adult giving a guest lecture. My adult ego state has to step in. As we all move through life, different situations and people will activate different ego states in us.

Importantly, ego states don't exist in isolation. They are relational, meaning that in order to exist, they require someone else to interact with and have emotional reactions to. These can be divided into complementary and crossed transactions.

Complementary transactions

A complementary transaction occurs when one person's ego state aligns with the desired ego state of another. A complementary transaction doesn't necessarily mean that the same ego states are involved, nor does *complementary* necessarily indicate that the interaction is good or desirable. For instance, in a marriage, one partner may constantly need nurturing and reassurance, refusing to take on household responsibilities and requiring pampering. This partner is in a child ego state. The other partner may adopt a parental ego state, providing care, making decisions, and nurturing the first partner. Both partners might be content with this arrangement: one enjoys being cared for, while the other finds fulfilment in being nurturing. Their transactions complement each other's ego states.

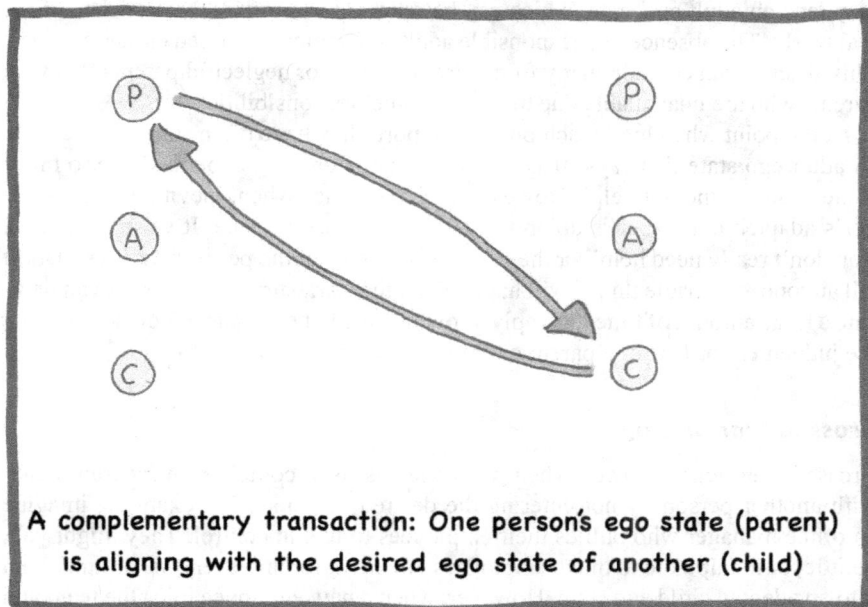

A complementary transaction: One person's ego state (parent) is aligning with the desired ego state of another (child)

However, over time, problems may arise. The nurturing partner may feel trapped and resentful because their childlike partner depends on them for everything, while the dependent partner might feel restricted and helpless.

Male survivors of abuse may recognise a complementary transaction with their abuser, regardless of their age at the time of the abuse. Abusers often adopt a parent ego state to control their victim. Some use a critical parent ego state, being threatening or aggressive and saying things like, 'You should know it upsets me and I get nasty when you behave like that.' Others may use a nurturing parent ego state, encouraging intimacy with phrases like, 'Come on, let me show you how much I love you'. Both approaches attempt to manoeuvre the victim into an adapted child ego state, making them compliant and willing to please.

Even after the abuse has stopped, survivors often carry the adapted child within them and may internalise the abuser's parent ego state. They can relive the abusive dynamic internally, hearing both their abuser's and their own voices, although the abuser's voice is often much louder. Societal attitudes towards male survivors, which often diminish their voices, can perpetuate this dynamic. As a result, survivors may remain in a complementary transactional relationship with their abuser long after the abuse has ended. Interestingly, there is a conspicuous absence of an adult ego state in most survivor–perpetrator interactions. Perpetrators rarely, if ever, occupy an authentic adult ego state, which would require them to confront the impact of their actions. Abuse is so powerful that the survivor is rarely able to neutrally process the experience, particularly when it is ongoing; therefore, they, too, often go without an adult ego state. Survivors who were abused in childhood or adolescence, may lack an adult ego state, which can be reflected in survivors' experience of the real world. The absence of a responsible adult is common in abused children's lives. This absence can come in many forms, from abusive or neglectful parents to loving parents who are unavailable due to work or other responsibilities.

At the point when men reach out for support, they have often started to develop an adult ego state that says, 'Right, this has gone on long enough. Time to make some changes and get help'. However, a battle comes when, inevitably, the survivor's adapted child speaks up and says, 'Don't cause a scene. It wasn't that bad. You don't really need help', or the internalised voice of the perpetrator says, 'Don't tell anyone, or terrible things will happen'. At the start, survivors' therapy can dedicate a huge amount of time to simply allowing an adult ego state to develop without the judgement or fear of a parent or child ego state.

Crossed transaction

Crossed transactions occur when someone resists a complementary transaction with another person by not entering the desired ego state. For example, imagine an office manager who bullies their employees to feel in control. They might yell, belittle, or manipulate to make employees obedient, forcing everyone around them into an adapted child ego state. However, when a new employee joins the team and sees this unacceptable behaviour, they might refuse to go into an adapted child ego state, instead remaining in an adult ego state. They may calmly say, 'You can't treat people this way' and complain to HR. This is a crossed transaction.

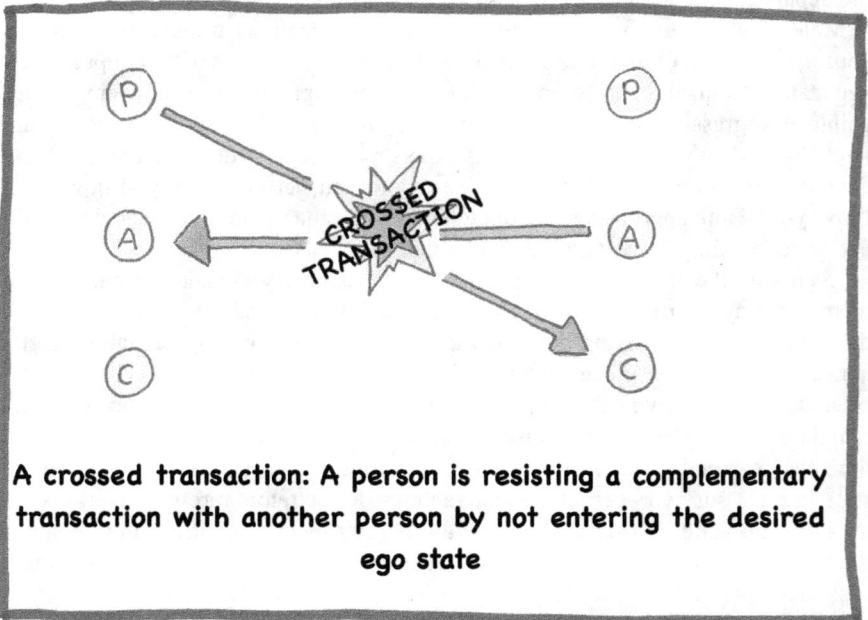

A crossed transaction: A person is resisting a complementary transaction with another person by not entering the desired ego state

I often see male survivors at the transition point from a complementary transaction with a perpetrator, in which they keep the perpetrator's secrets, feel shamed, and live in the shadow of abuse, to a crossed transaction, in which they no longer want to be under the influence of the abuser and disclose the abuse or seek help or justice. Often, this happens years after the abuse, after some event in the survivor's life – be it the birth of a child, the death of a perpetrator, or reaching a significant milestone (eg, a birthday, retirement, etc) – makes the survivor want to change their relationship with the perpetrator.

Complementary and crossed transactions happen across societies. A dominant group might try to control a minority group, for instance, by making laws that disproportionately impact that group. The dominant group expects the minority group to comply by being the adapted child, creating a complementary transaction. But if the group resists and fights back, it creates a crossed transaction.

6.2   Orphaning ourselves from biological family

I've spent countless hours discussing with survivors the dilemma of cutting ties with family members. Those considering this step often feel like lone satellites circling around a planet (their family) that's filled with toxic gases. Sometimes, events like holidays or birthdays pull the satellite closer to the family's orbit. Survivors may temporarily leave the safety of their satellite and land on the planet's surface, only to be overwhelmed by its poisonous atmosphere and retreating to their isolation. Some survivors don't even have a satellite to retreat to; they're stuck on the planet's surface, unable to break free from the gravitational pull. They remain in the toxic environment, suffocating and lacking personal space. Many survivors find themselves trapped in this dynamic for years, and often, the only thing that brings relief is a big event, like leaving for work or university or the death of a problematic family member.

Orphaning yourself

For some people, the idea of cutting off families and fundamentally orphaning themselves is out of the question. They think of it as a counterintuitive and shameful concept that they never consider. They stay connected to their families without ever questioning whether they should. For survivors of sexual abuse, this can have serious consequences. It can keep us connected to those who abused us, people who failed to protect us then, and people who fail to support us now. Not only that, but as we age, we may feel an increasing responsibility or pressure to take care of those people. We can feel desperately lonely when we are tied to a family who failed us. Following are some common reasons survivors stay in contact with families or family members who cause them pain or whom they want to cut off.

Social expectations

Many cultures value prioritising family above everything else. This expectation can be particularly pronounced for men, who may feel additional burdens to provide for and protect family members. The expectation of a relationship with our family can be so strong that it discourages authentic conversations about whether the relationship is healthy for us.

Fear of being alone

Many male survivors of sexual abuse know what it is to feel alone. For some, family may be one of the only sources of consistent human contact. Even if our families make us feel bad or treat us with disrespect, the fear that we would be alone without them can be so strong that we keep them in our lives, despite the damage it may do to us.

Cultural ties

Family, cultural, and social ties are interlinked for many survivors, particularly those in ethnic minority communities. Those who attend a mosque, church, or synagogue in order to connect to their cultural, social, and religious community may also have contact with family or friends of family there. When we share these sorts of spaces with our family or are part of a close community who expects us to honour our family, regardless of circumstances, this can make it more difficult to separate from them.

Feelings of responsibility, duty, or guilt

No matter how self-aware we are, all of us are vulnerable to feeling pressure to meet societal expectations of right and wrong. This can create a sense of obligation to put our feelings aside and care for families who may not have ever cared for us. On top of this, we often experience direct pressure from friends or family. People might say, 'You should speak to your dad more', without realising how painful that is for us.

Some family members feel entitled to contact us because they looked after us at one time or gave birth to us, and they may communicate this by making us feel like we owe them access to us, regardless of whether we want to give it. Sexual abuse is all about taking advantage and disregarding boundaries. Family members who guilt us into caring for them are not violating us in the same way as sexual abuse, but their behaviour *is* another attempt to compromise our boundaries and make us do things we know we do not want to do.

Reliance on family for support

Some men, despite relying on family for support, may also find the option of orphaning ourselves desirable. This reliance may result from financial support or having a caring role in the survivor's life, particularly for survivors with learning or physical disabilities. These relationships can become codependent, built on practical as well as emotional support.

Young survivors in their teens or early twenties, too, might need to live at home or rely on family members. This can become more complicated if the young person lives with the perpetrator or in a family that facilitated the abuse. The young person might also be a member of a sexual minority group – a trans, bi, or gay man, for example – in a family who would discriminate against him. Young people in such circumstances often hide part of their authentic selves while managing the aftermath of sexual abuse by themselves.

Other survivors have caring responsibilities for family members. We may love a family member very much and willingly care for them, but be required, as a result, to stay connected with other family members who are harmful, abusive, or have some other negative impact on our lives.

Hope for healing that doesn't come

Some survivors feel torn between wanting to orphan ourselves and wanting to be close to family. We take small crumbs of attention that feel good and make that good feeling go far. For example, if one in ten family visits goes well, this gives us hope. Many survivors have an inner child inside us that hopes for a healing experience. Even though we are adults, we still carry the emotional needs of our childhood selves in our hearts, and we desperately try to get family to meet those needs. Occasionally we might see our family and have it go well. We may think, *Maybe this is getting easier*, or *They are changing*, only to be disappointed when things go wrong. We may feel abandoned or disrespected, our inner child neglected all over again. Some of us stay in this behaviour pattern for years, looking for a healing experience that makes what happened to us as children better, even when we know that will never happen.

Each survivor who has a difficult relationship with their family will need to come to their own conclusions about maintaining those relationships or orphaning themselves. There is no easy way to decide what it is right for you, and there are few opportunities to discuss the possibilities. However, according to Stand Alone, a UK charity working with adults who are vulnerable and estranged from their families, at least five million people in the UK have chosen to stop contact with a family member.[1]

Reflective activity

If you're struggling to set boundaries with family, here are some questions you might ask yourself about whether you want to cut family off or not. You can consider them by yourself, take them to a friend, or work through them with a therapist. There are no right or wrong answers; these questions are about you figuring out what is best for you right now. You can always change your mind in the future.

- Are you considering cutting ties altogether, or could you renegotiate the terms of your relationship? For instance, you might see the person less often or in less demanding situations.
- Have you thought about reframing your perspective on family? Instead of relying on them for emotional support or love, could you view them as friends, with lower expectations?
- Do you feel emotionally and physically safe around your family? If not, why subject yourself to harm? If this is a recurring pattern, what drives you to put yourself in vulnerable situations? Can this pattern be altered?
- If you opt to sever ties, how can you establish support systems for yourself?

Take time with these questions. You might pick the ones that are most useful and discuss them with a friend or therapist to get different perspectives.

For some survivors, family is a crucial, at times, even a lifesaving source of support. However, if you're among those who don't feel safe, supported, or adequately equipped by their family to recover from abuse, it's important to explore other sources of support. Many people seek support beyond their biological families, forming new nurturing bonds with individuals who understand and support them in a profound way. This practice has come known as finding a 'chosen family'.

6.3   Chosen family

We are often told that blood is thicker than water, meaning that biological ties to family are more important than any other relationship we might form. However, did you know that this saying is a misquote? The original saying, 'The blood of the covenant is thicker than the water of the womb', is an English proverb that dates back to medieval times, and the meaning has shifted over the centuries. Historically, the saying actually meant the complete opposite of the modern phrase. The original proverb meant that the bonds created through experience, agreements, and conscious decisions are more meaningful than those that are obligated through familial bonds.

It can be a relief all by itself for some survivors whose family harmed them to know the true meaning of this old proverb. It means that the so-called 'societal truth' that biological family should be our priority, regardless of the circumstances, is actually unfounded. For survivors who want to orphan themselves, freeing themselves from perceived social obligations can be the first step towards creating distance and forming a chosen family.

The term *chosen family* was coined by anthropologist Kath Weston in her 1991 book *Families We Choose: Lesbians, Gays, Kinship*. The book examines kinship among gay men and lesbians and how they form chosen family units built on love and friendship. Weston argues that these family groups can exist apart from and are just as important as the biological families LGBTQIA+ people grew up in.[2] Many examples exist of LGBTQIA+ people forming these important chosen families. During the AIDS crisis, many men dying of AIDS-related illnesses were rejected by both healthcare professionals and family members, leaving fellow LGBTQIA+ people responsible for their end-of-life care. This traumatic time created many chosen families between gay men, as well as lesbians, many of whom cared for dying friends and participated in activism that changed attitudes and policies towards people with HIV/AIDS.

Another example of chosen family is the ballroom community, a music and dance subculture created for and by LGBTQIA+ people and queer and trans people of colour (QTPOC). In ballroom communities, chosen families are represented by 'houses' led by 'mothers' and 'fathers' who provide care and support for the 'children' within that house. These houses compete with other houses in different dance and performance styles, the most well-known example of which is the dance style 'voguing'. Ballroom houses are no stranger to oppression and violence. Their earliest iteration may date back to the 1880s in the United States, where former slave William Dorsey Swann hosted secret balls and performed as a drag queen. He was arrested multiple times over his life, including for throwing parties with 'Black men in full elegant female costumes dancing to live drums, banjos, and fiddle'.[3]

Chosen families have been important for LGBTQIA+ folk throughout history, and the term is increasingly being embraced by other minoritised (care leavers, immigrants, disabled people, neurodivergent people, BDSM communities, etc) and stigmatised (male survivors) groups. The male survivor groups I run are often described by the men who attend them as one big extended family. I suspect this is because groups of male survivors often provide each other with space to be understood, to talk (or not talk) about their abuse, and to share humour, as well as coping strategies. These are key ingredients to creating a successful chosen family.

Not everyone will be able to access therapy groups or be willing to attend them. Some survivors may want a chosen family without having to disclose their abuse. Whatever type of chosen family feels right to you, here are seven points to consider when looking for your people.

1. What should my chosen family look like?

Many survivors fantasise about having a large group of friends. In reality, however, surviving sexual abuse may mean that large groups of people can be challenging. In therapy, I've heard many survivors wish they could thrive in groups, juggling different people with endless energy. But in truth, our ideal chosen family may not look like that. We might not be able to comfortably sit in large groups. We might do better with a chosen family made up of one, two, or three people. Thinking about what we want versus what we are able to maintain and nurture is important when looking for our chosen family.

2. Give it time

Finding your chosen family will take time. Many men struggle to find meaningful relationships. Heterosexual men often find themselves in social situations that don't allow them to speak honestly about their emotions or their desire to form close bonds with others. Gay men might have access to specifically gay spaces but may still feel marginalised in those spaces. Many LGBTQIA+ survivors say they do not feel 'gay enough' to be comfortable in those spaces or ask for their needs. Finding your chosen family will take time and require you to keep putting yourself out there. Often, this includes stepping out of your comfort zone.

3. Pay attention to your instincts

It is rare to identify a chosen family member straightaway, so allow your instincts to guide you. If someone feels nice but not right, don't try to force them into a relationship you'll both end up resenting. Look for people who make you feel good about yourself and your relationship. Find ways to nurture those friendships naturally, without rushing it. The process takes time, so focus on how you feel and where your comfort levels are.

4. Be explicit about your boundaries and what you want

It's no good replacing a harmful biological family for a chosen family that is harmful in different ways. Make sure to communicate your boundaries and expectations. Stating your intentions and what makes you uncomfortable allows people to meet your expectations and communicate where they need compromise. Being explicit about what you want upfront will also help you spot people who may not be compatible with what you want, and this can save you energy and disappointment.

5. Check in with your new family

Checking in can be a main difference between a friendship group and a chosen family. People within friendship groups, regardless of how close they are, will also have families that check in with them and support them. For those in a chosen family, this might not be the case; the members of a chosen family check in with each other. Check-ins don't have to be heavy or time-consuming; they simply need to communicate that you are thinking of the other person and open up the opportunity to talk, if it is needed.

6.   Try not to sacrifice too much

All new relationships require compromise. It is an important part of what keep social groups functioning. But compromise can be a delicate thing to get right. Try to keep in mind the bigger picture: sacrificing some of your needs is okay if you're getting what you need overall, because it is likely that other chosen family members are making similar sacrifices. However, when we have painful experiences like abuse, we may be tempted to sacrifice all of our needs to make relationships work. Keep evaluating whether you are compromising too much. If you are, talk about it with the other person. If that doesn't work, don't be afraid to walk away from a chosen family group that doesn't meet your needs.

7.   Risk vulnerability

This may be the hardest one, and it reflects another difference between a friendship group and a chosen family. While many friendships involve vulnerability, many others never get beyond surface level. A chosen family consists of people who accept your vulnerability and support you. It might not be appropriate or comfortable to open up about your abuse or problematic family at first, but at some point, it is necessary to take the risk of being vulnerable. It is absolutely a risk – there is no way of sugar coating that – but the reward could be finding a chosen family who listens to you and makes you feel heard and understood in a way your biological family was not able to do. For ideas about how to talk to a chosen family about your abuse, see Chapter 9, 'Disclosure'.

I am aware that many men feel that their social circle is small. You might feel completely alone or that stepping out of your comfort zone to seek a chosen family is overwhelming or impractical. This is a process, and it takes trial and error and continuous effort. It can feel exhausting, so remember to pace yourself and take little steps. You won't find a chosen family overnight; even if you throw everything at it, it still takes time.

You might try looking for events that people with similar hobbies might attend or finding existing interest groups. You won't walk away from every event or group meeting with a new friend, but that is okay. Practising being in these types of spaces can help you feel a little more comfortable each time you do it. Even if the thought of small talk fills you with dread, it can help to view it like a muscle you need to work out. Exercise it often, and you'll start to find others with shared interests who might, with time, become family.

Managing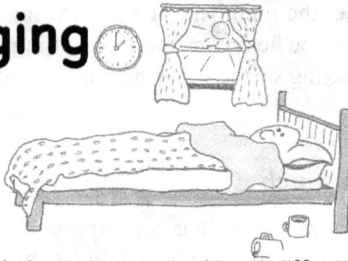

Depression

Depression can drain our energy, making it difficult to engage in even the activities we once enjoyed. This often leads to decreased activity, which can intensify feelings of depression. However, breaking this cycle is possible. Even small steps toward being active can make a meaningful difference in improving mood and well-being. Try these three steps:

① **Choose activities you are likely to complete**	• **Exercise:** Try anything from getting around the local park, stretches in your chair to weightlifting or swimming • **Socialise:** Call or message a friend, organise a dinner, visit family, join a club / group • **Responsibilities:** Tidy your home, look into professional development courses, do DIY • **Hobbies:** Try sports, gardening, drawing, playing music, hiking, playing with a pet, cooking • **Self-care:** Get a haircut or make a healthy meal
② **Practice your chosen activities**	• **Start small:** Take breaks and don't over commit to a new activity • **Make a plan:** Don't leave it to the last minute, plan your activity • **Bring a friend:** Arrange to do your activity with someone
③ **Social Support**	• **Connect:** Prioritise connecting with loved ones in person or remotely–try a video call to cook together, play a video game, or share a coffee over the phone • **Agree to socialising:** Say yes to seeing people • **Reach out:** Find formal help, either therapy or a support group

Use this space to list activities you could try to help manage depression:

www.jeremysachs.com   @JeremySachs_

For A4 and printable versions of this worksheet, visit www.jeremysachs.com

For A4 and printable versions of this worksheet, visit www.jeremysachs.com

Resources

Games People Play *by Eric Berne*

ISBN 0140027688
This is the original book on TA. It aims to help readers understand relationships and our role in them. It was successful at the time of its publication in 1964 and continues to be hugely influential. Apparently, Kurt Vonnegut was a fan of the book, and it allegedly inspired country singer Conway Twitty's song 'Games People Play'.

Families We Choose: Lesbians, Gays, Kinship *by Kath Weston*

ISBN: 9780231110938
This is the original book on chosen families. It draws on fieldwork and interviews to bring to life different experiences of kinship among gay men and lesbians.

Pose *(2018–2021)*

Set in the late 1980s and early 1990s, this television series focuses on the lives of Black and Latino LGBTQ+ communities and their 'houses', where chosen families provide support and compete in ballroom competitions. The show also addresses issues such as the AIDS crisis and trans rights.

Signposting

Tavistock Relationships

https://tavistockrelationships.org
This therapy centre provides excellent training for therapists, as well as inclusive relationship therapy. I occasionally lecture there and have found them to be inclusive and well trauma-informed.

Relate

www.relate.org.uk, www.relationships-scotland.org.uk
Relate provides couples' therapy throughout England and Scotland.

Mental Health Foundation

www.mentalhealth.org.uk
This organisation works to promote good mental health for all, including men who have experienced trauma. They provide resources and run campaigns focused on better mental health.

Notes

1 'The prevalence of family estrangement', Stand Alone, 2014. www.standalone.org. uk/wp-content/uploads/2013/08/StandAlonePrevalenceRESEARCH3.pdf, accessed 3 June 2024.
2 Kath Weston, *Families We Choose: Lesbians, Gays, Kinship* (New York: Columbia University Press, 1991).
3 Otis Alexander, 'William Dorsey Swann (1858–1954)', BlackPast.org, updated 7 November 2023. www.blackpast.org/african-american-history/william-dorsey-swann-1858-1954, accessed 3 June 2024.

Chapter 7

Sex, gender, and nurturing our authentic Sexual Self

Chapter Contents

I've never met my true self

I was abused by three different men between the ages of 6 and 17. Firstly by a man who lived in the flat beneath ours, then a teacher, and lastly by a family relative. The relative was a one-off, while the others happened more times than I remember. Back when I was a boy, men had to be tough, I grew up in a certain part of East London where you couldn't show any weakness, and yet, I was walking around with the shame of being a victim to these men. I know now I tried to overcompensate. I would fight anyone who looked at me the wrong way, which is why the abuse felt extra shameful... if I could handle myself in the streets, why did I just let the abuse happen to me?

Looking back now, I realise I couldn't be mates with men. Or if I could, fighting or drugs or drink had to be involved. To me, men were either a threat or something I needed to dominate. Since I retired from the post office, I'm starting to understand I'm uncomfortable around men because of the abuse, but also I feel attracted to them. I can't bring myself to label it yet. I know it's called bisexual, but I have never ever said that word. I flinched the first time a therapist said it to me; I felt physically sick. I know the world has changed and I guess it's my job to try and change with it. I joined a support group and met gay men. I really get on with them, but after, I beat myself up because I also still feel disgust at myself. I'm old now, so I don't know what to do with this, I don't know whether I'll ever want to express this side of my Sexual Self. At the moment, I'm working on just being sober and being

DOI: 10.4324/9781003423331-7

friends with other men – they don't have to be a threat. Maybe one day I'll meet someone but who knows, I'm taking it day by day.

George, aged 68, working class

7.1   The rupturing of our Sexual Self: Abuse in childhood, adolescence, and adulthood

Western society is good at talking about sex. The trouble is, it's good at talking about it in ways that are defensive, shaming, binary, fictionalised, or comedic. Examples exist throughout history of non-Western cultures that expressed sexuality and gender differently. Sadly, they are often overlooked or forgotten by Western audiences, thanks to the immense impact of colonialism. This means that survivors are often left with very few ways to think about our sexuality or gender outside masculine stereotypes within a strict binary. These cultural restrictions, alongside the experience of abuse, can make it difficult to get into contact with our Sexual Self. The term *Sexual Self* was first used by psychiatrist Avodah Offit in the 1980s to describe how our personalities and character can affect our sexuality.[1] Since then, the phrase has taken on a life of its own. It is used to describe not only people's experience during sex, but also how they feel about sex, their sexuality and what sex means to them.

Societal pressures and sexual abuse can cause us to keep our Sexual Self hidden deep down within us. We may feel uncomfortable, awkward, or even retraumatised when discussing it. While some survivors have no problem being flirty or joking about sex with friends, on dates, or on dating apps, they may lose confidence or freeze when it comes to expressing their authentic Sexual Self.

Our authentic Sexual Self can begin with natural play and exploration when we are young children. Children under five have little or no inhibition about being naked, can show curiosity about other people's bodies and enjoy talking about bodily functions using words like *poo* or *wee*. As they grow, they role-play adult relationships. They do this commonly with the children of close family friends, cousins, or best friends at school. Games like 'boyfriend and girlfriend' or 'mummy and daddy', are acted out. Gender also gets experimentation in fancy dress games and fantasy. Behaviours like hand-holding, kissing on the cheek, clothes swapping, and using a parent's clothes or makeup are common. As children get older, this develops into what we recognise as sexual behaviour and gender expression. Teenagers make sexual jokes, express themselves through music, makeup, or clothing, seek relationships, experiment with sexuality and gender, explore their own bodies, and masturbate. By the end of adolescence, the Sexual Self has solidified. While it can still change in adulthood, it doesn't go through such dramatic growth as it did in childhood and teenage years. Often, these formative years lay crucial foundations for our Sexual Self and how we express it.

Many teens and adults have a limited vocabulary for sexually intimate or vulnerable situations. Our language can feel reduced down to 'Yes'/'No' and 'I like that'/'I don't like that'. In some cases, we may not even have these few words, desperately wishing sexual partners could read our minds to know what we do or don't want. In other cases, particularly for abuse survivors, our Sexual Self may disappear completely, leaving us in sexual situations where our only choices are fight, flight, or freeze (see Chapter 2, page 28).

The Sexual Self is unique to each individual, and the effect of sexual abuse on it can be just as unique. It would be impossible to catalogue or summarise every impact sexual abuse has had on your Sexual Self and your relationship with sex, sexuality, and gender. However, the following subsections are intended to reflect some of the ways abuse can affect us depending on whether it occurs in childhood, adolescence, or adulthood. This isn't a hierarchy. It isn't better to be abused at one age than another, and there is no competition of suffering. It simply illustrates some potential impacts on the Sexual Self that may occur based on when you experienced the abuse. This does not mean that if you were abused in childhood, you will not relate to the experiences of those abused in adulthood and vice versa.

Before you read these subsections, I want to invite you to check in with how you are feeling. Regardless of whether you're a survivor or an ally, this subject has the potential to take us back to times when we were vulnerable. Reading about childhood or teenage years can transport us right back there. Thinking about abuse in adulthood can amplify those voices in our heads that shout, 'We should have fought back!' or 'Why did we put ourselves in that situation?' Remember to take care of yourself. We can be tempted to read about sex and abuse quickly to try and make sense of how we feel. But speed doesn't always help. This book will be here tomorrow. Take your time and be kind to yourself.

Childhood

For those of us who experience sexual abuse before an emergent sexuality, in pre-pubescence (childhood), abuse can make no sense. Children have not begun to think about sex or see their bodies in a way that adults would consider sexual. They have not started any part of their sexual development beyond natural play and exploration with their peers of the same age. Abuse at this stage means a child's emergent sexuality is impacted from the very beginning. This can cause difficulties because we enter adolescence and adulthood not knowing what our sexual identity would have been or how it would have developed without the experience of abuse. As adults, we not only must come to terms with our history of sexual abuse, but we may also start the journey to know our Sexual Self much later in life, without the benefit of childhood safety, experimentation, or play. An example of this is discovering sexuality. I have worked with men who have lived heterosexual lives, marrying women and having children, and never found the space to consider any other way of being. When they join a therapy group or begin therapy, however, they start to question whether early abuse robbed them of the safety to experiment, date outside of typical gender norms, or question what their Sexual Self may really want.

A child's brain may deal with abuse in different ways. It may push the abuse down and try to forget it. It's common for adults who survived different types of abuse or ACEs in childhood to have few or no memories of being a child. In other cases of abuse in early life, children can become prematurely sexualised and may replicate sex acts they have experienced with other children. These situations, in which a child is both a victim and an abuser, are often complicated, and the adults around them may willingly ignore this behaviour, putting it down to developmentally appropriate play or experimentation. Neither the prematurely sexualised child nor the victim may be able to tell the difference until later in life.

Adolescence

Sexual abuse in puberty (adolescence) occurs when a person's sense of sexuality is emerging. Adolescents have moved out of childlike experimentation and play and are starting to develop an active interest in sex. This is a delicate time in the development of the psyche and Sexual Self, and abuse can trample over it, not allowing sexuality to develop appropriately or in its own time. This can be particularly isolating because Western society often expects sexual development and experimentation from teenagers. Attitudes assuming that teenage boys are 'lucky' to have sex or that 'boys will be boys' are common (particularly when the perpetrator is female), when in fact, teenagers may be engaged in unhealthy or unsafe sexual behaviours. These assumptions also leave teenage boys particularly vulnerable to coercive sexual abuse or grooming, as the signs of sexual abuse are less likely to be noticed when observers assume boys are actively expressing their sexuality.

Some survivors who had sexual experiences at this age have no doubt in their minds that they were abused. For others, however, it isn't as clear. During puberty, our emergent sexuality means we are just starting to get to know our Sexual Self. At the same time, we are still vulnerable, drawn to parents, parental figures, and peers who we feel understand us. It can be confusing if someone who occupies an important, understanding role in our lives abuses us. Many survivors grapple with our experience, wondering if the sexual contact was abuse at all. In these cases, I encourage survivors to think about the power dynamic between themselves and the abuser. Even if we feel powerful as teenagers, most adults around us have significant power over us. If your experience doesn't feel right and you can look back and recognise a power imbalance, chances are there was some sort of abuse happening.

Adulthood

Abuse can also happen in adulthood, after we have a developed sense of sexuality. This abuse can shatter a secure Sexual Self, as well as a sense of safety in the broader world. It can destroy previously safe relationships with loved ones, work, and the world. Abuse in adulthood can lead to self-criticising or self-punishing voices in our heads. We can punish ourselves for our actions leading up to the abuse (eg, *Why did I go to that club/drink too much/trust that person?*). We can also criticise ourselves for not taking action during the abuse (eg, *Why didn't I run away/fight back?*).

The experience of being a man abused as an adult is underrepresented in support services, therapy rooms, and society. This can make it an isolating and shameful experience, leaving us to ourselves with self-criticising and self-punishing voices going around and around in our minds without support or help.

Across different ages

It's common to find that men who were sexually abused in childhood encounter further abuse later in life. Often, this is because such men have often grown up in an environment that exposed them to a greater risk of harm: if you were at risk of abuse in childhood, chances are your environment did not get safer in adolescence and early adulthood. The effect of environment on abuse demonstrates the importance of understanding intersectional issues, both for survivors working to understand ourselves and our history and for professionals trying to understand each survivor's unique experience. Sexual abuse in early life can be so disturbing that male survivors become drawn to risky behaviours. To soothe the profound pain of traumatic memories (both conscious and unconscious), we may turn to destructive behaviour such as drug-taking, excessive drinking, infidelity, or risky sex. While it is important not to make moral judgements on these behaviours, which can be attempts to handle the pain of trauma, it is useful to acknowledge that some coping strategies can have a detrimental impact on our lives, which can include exposing ourselves to others who look for vulnerable people to abuse.

The Sexual Self often needs emotional and physical safety in order to develop authentically and enable us to seek connections with others who are also emotionally and physically safe. Sexual abuse at any age can disrupt our feeling of safety. Our Sexual Self retreats deep within us to avoid being damaged. It can hide so well that we may find we have no idea how to find it again.

The Sexual Self is almost always negatively impacted by sexual abuse. What that impact looks like can vary. In fact, different people can appear to have completely opposite reactions to abuse. Some people may want to abstain from sex completely, avoiding anything to do with it. Often, this leads them to feel isolated and lonely. Others might feel driven towards sex, seeking it out at the cost of loving relationships or putting themselves in unsafe situations. Despite their differences, these opposite behaviours and feelings are common responses rooted in similar experiences of abuse. In the following section, I describe several painful sexual behaviours that male survivors of sexual abuse may recognise.

7.2   Sexual behaviours that cause pain

Sex is at the heart of our identity. We can spend a lifetime learning about our Sexual Self and what it means to us. We learn what we like, what we don't like, who we want to have sex with and how. Even if we are asexual or decide to not make sex a big part of our identity, sex is still everywhere. We have to navigate a society constantly pushing heteronormative and simplistic ideas about sex. It is no wonder that when our Sexual Self becomes damaged, other parts of our life start to unravel as well. We can feel unmanly for not wanting sex, as if we don't live up to expectations of what a man should be. Alternatively, we can feel possessed by sex to the point it interferes with everyday life. This can have an impact on our partner, too. We can desire sexual gratification so much that we lead a double life separate from our partner, keeping secrets from them. Or we may detach from our Sexual Self, becoming numb to sexual desire. Our partner despairs, begging us to have sex when we don't know how to start.

Some survivors may desire sex so much that it feels like an addiction, a 'fix' we need to satisfy something deep within us before getting on with our life – until the next time an urge for sex comes along. The term *sex addiction* can be useful to survivors describing this experience. Preoccupation with sex or sexual relief can feel comparable to the need to take drugs or have a drink. Although unlike drugs and alcohol that stop being pleasurable, this does not necessarily occur with sex. Of course, sex or orgasming to help regulate trauma symptoms isn't inherently bad, but if survivors only have the one strategy of sex to manage the distress, then sex can become difficult to manage and feel addictive.

However, I'm hesitant to use the terms *sex addiction* and *sex addict* for a number of reasons. First, a number of powerful public figures have used the term *sex addiction* as an excuse for their abusive behaviour. Since the #MeToo era, many high-profile people have been publicly revealed to have exploited their power and position in order to coerce, abuse, or rape people of all genders over whom they have power. When they are caught and prosecuted, several have used 'sex addiction' as a way of justifying their abusive behaviour. This defence tries to shift the focus away from the people who were victimised, ignores the gross power imbalance involved, and frames the perpetrator as a victim. Second, while new research is emerging all the time, findings can often be contradictory, and there remains a lack of clinical research in the field of sex addiction. While many books and resources on sex addiction are out there, it's not a recognised mental health diagnosis in the *Diagnostic and Statistical Manual of Mental Disorders, 5th edition* (DSM-5). The WHO's *International Classification of Disease, 11th revision* (ICD-11) includes the clinical term *compulsive sexual behaviour disorder*, which is classified as an impulse control disorder, rather than an addiction.[2] Even this is controversial, as the ICD-11's diagnosis failed its first reliability test in an international published study in the *Journal of Behavioral Addictions*. The study showed that only 50 per cent of mental health professionals diagnosed it correctly, while others misdiagnosed it due to personal bias.[3] The third reason for my hesitance to use the term *sex addict* is that it is often used against survivors who behave in any way outside the sexual norms of their community. Some partners or family members weaponise the term, using it to express disgust or legitimise their own moral outrage, often using non-evidence-based sources to back them up. I've sat with many men whose partner has called them a sex addict after they attempted to talk about ethical non-monogamy, kink, sexuality, compulsive sex, or frequency of sex within the relationship. Weaponisation of the term *sex addict* is one more way male survivors can be oppressed by our family, religious community, or society's moral judgements.

Ultimately, the language you choose to describe your experience of sex is yours. It may change as your relationship with sex changes, or it may not. For the purposes of this book, I will use the term *compulsive sexual behaviour* when describing some forms of sex that can cause us pain. I trust you to apply what's in these pages to your own experience, regardless of whether we choose to use the same language.

Following are some common issues survivors bring up when it comes to sex and intimacy. If you struggle with sex, you might recognise your behaviour in more than one of these categories. This doesn't make you strange or deviant; it makes you human. In fact, many people not affected by sexual abuse might also look at this list and recognise their behaviour. Most of us desire sex and sexual connection, and it can become difficult for multiple reasons, not least because, as I noted at the beginning of this chapter, authentic conversations about sex are rare. However sexual abuse can make these issues louder, more pronounced. and more laced with shame.

Compulsive sexual behaviour

The ICD-11 describes compulsive sexual behaviour disorder as 'characterised by a persistent pattern of failure to control intense, repetitive sexual impulses or urges resulting in repetitive sexual behaviour'. The description goes on to add that this disorder can have a big impact on a person's life, potentially causing 'significant impairment in personal, family, social, educational, occupational, or other important areas of functioning'. Interestingly, the ICD-11 does not indicate how much sex is 'too much'; rather, it focuses on the emotional effect compulsive behaviour has on us rather than the nature or frequency of the sex.[4]

If you recognise your experience here, it does not mean you have a disorder; remember the research initially that found only 50 per cent of healthcare professionals diagnosed compulsive sexual disorder correctly. This chapter is not about diagnosing you. More and more, we are learning that diagnoses for mental health issues exist on a spectrum rather than as a tick-box exercise. Absolutely, you may sit further along the spectrum than other people in your life, but this does not mean you have a disorder. Even if you did, that would be okay. The quotes from the ICD-11 are meant to illustrate that this behaviour is well known and experienced by lots of people. You are not alone.

Compulsive sexual behaviour can manifest differently, depending on the individual. Following are some examples.

Online or digital sex

Online or digital sex can include lots of different behaviours. Some examples include

- Watching or collecting pornography from the internet
- Spending money on membership websites that host exclusive pornography content
- Spending hours finding people to sext online, in chatrooms or on social media or apps
- Paying for online sexual content from sex workers via websites like OnlyFans or Fansly
- Flirting with colleagues or friends via email or messaging services
- Desiring digisexual relationships – online sex and relationships that feel more satisfying and more fulfilling than in-person sex and relationships.

For men with various identities, online sex can be a preferred way of seeking sexual gratification. Trans men and men who are at higher risk of violence may feel safer online than they do in clubs, bars, or at sex parties where others might feel safe. However, online sex can come with its own risks. The online world can bring vulnerable people into contact with online perpetrators, which can compound previous sexual trauma or lead to a person's first exposure to abusive behaviour. Additionally, I want to be clear, these behaviours may be non-problematic for people if it does not impair the rest of life. Indeed, some men may spend hours on pornography and stay efficient at work, meeting all their life's responsibilities.

Some men, however, find their online world can become hypersexualised, leading them to take any and all chances for online sexual encounters, either via pornography or with strangers. This can feel like a double life, with the real world sustaining intimate and meaningful relationships and the online world sustaining anonymous, dark, and sexual ones. While this double-life behaviour is common in many men, LGBTQIA+ people can be particularly vulnerable to it. Online sex can be fun, and some people can sustain this type of double life with no problem while others find it prevents sex with partners or perpetuates stereotypes that can be difficult to live up to and cause shame if there's a history of sexual abuse.

Online sex can become a catalyst for new sexual behaviours or fixations. Men may be exposed to and seek out experiences they may never have known about had it not been for the internet. Online sex can escalate rapidly or gradually, from looking at videos and pictures to paying for online content or seeking risky sex in the real world. The sheer speed at which men can lose money to websites or develop new sexual focuses can be alarming. Part of the reason for this speed is online sex's broad accessibility through laptops, phones, and platforms like dating or anonymous chat apps, instant messaging platforms, and chat rooms.

Chemsex

Chemsex (older terms include party n' play [PnP] or high and horny [H&H]) is a term, used mostly among men who have sex with men, that describes the act of deliberately having sex under the influence of drugs. Rather than taking drugs or drinking and happening to have sex, in chemsex, people take drugs for the purpose of enhancing sexual activities.

Commonly used drugs are

- **GHB (gamma-hydroxybutyrate) and GBL (gamma butyrolactone).** Colloquial names include G, Gina, liquid ecstasy, X, liquid X, 'grievous bodily harm'. GHB and GBL are depressants that come in the form of a powder or clear liquid. It can cause euphoria, leading users to lose inhibitions and gain confidence. The drug can be difficult to dose, as even taking slightly too much can send users 'under', leading them to become unconscious and unresponsive. It's common for men using GHB to pre-dose or measure out doses before heading to a party or event where there will be sex. GBL is a precursor to GHB, which means that it is converted to GHB inside the body after swallowing.
- **Crystal meth (methamphetamine).** Colloquial names include Tina, T, ice. Crystal meth is a powerful drug that comes in either powder, tablets, or crystals. It can be snorted (bumped), swallowed (bombed), injected (slammed), or smoked. It can lower inhibitions, increase energy, and suppress appetite. It can also increase sexual desire, which can lead users to behave in risky ways.
- **Meth (mephedrone).** Colloquial names include M, M-cat, meow meow, plant food. Meth is similar to speed and ecstasy, which are all amphetamines, and comes in a fine white or yellowish powder or as crystallised granules. It is snorted or swallowed in tablet form or powder wrapped in paper or rizla paper. It causes euphoria, making users feel alert, confident, and talkative.

All three of these drugs have stimulant properties that enhance sexual arousal. They are taken in combination and culminate in sex or sexual sessions that last over an extended period of time and may involve a number of sexual partners. Additionally, some survivors have told me that they may use these drugs solo to stay home and masturbate. Other drugs used to a lesser extent in chemsex include cocaine and ketamine.

Chemsex has a complicated relationship with sexual abuse. Chemsex environments can be difficult to navigate, and participants' capacity to ask for or give consent is often impaired. Sexual abuse may occur in a chemsex environment when users do not pay attention to whether other participants have 'gone under' and are not able to consent. In some cases, men report being deliberately dosed with GHB without their knowledge to enable sexual abuse or other crimes (like robbery). Chemsex environments also come with the risk of sexuality transmitted illnesses (STIs). In the UK, the 2020 introduction of pre-exposure prophylaxis (PrEP) in the NHS reduced the risk of contracting HIV in chemsex environments, but some risk of HIV persists, and other STIs continue to be a danger in these environments.

Despite the risks, some survivors are drawn to chemsex environments. Survivors have shared with me that taking part in chemsex can be cathartic and even therapeutic. Glenn, a guest on a chemsex episode of my podcast, talked about its appeal:

> It's escapism. So it's escapism from the pain of sexual abuse in childhood, but also, years later, when both my parents became ill and eventually died, there was the stress around the loss of parents, so chems and sex, and chemsex was useful in getting over that. There's also the idea that chemsex is somehow wrong, what happened to me as a child was wrong, as an adult I ran away from my past by doing something wrong and illegal.
>
> Both the abuse and the chemsex were taboo. Combining gay sex, which in some parts of the world is discriminated against ... with Class-A drugs actually gave me a feeling of power. ... [I]t enabled me to put two fingers up at society. It was, 'I don't care what people think. I'm going to do this'. But in the end, it was, 'I don't care what happens to me'.[5]

For some survivors who feel strong sexual compulsions, the chemsex environment can be perfect to feed a sexual appetite that feels out of control. For some survivors, it also gives opportunities to act out shame, punishing themselves with excessive drug-taking behaviours, abusing their body with drugs, a lack of sleep and nutrients, and sexually risky behaviour and revictimisation.

However, every man who takes part in chemsex has different reasons for seeking it out. It's problematic to assume all people who engage in chemsex do it from a place of trauma or abuse. Many have fun experiences and may even find the opportunities to learn new things about their Sexual Self. It's important for peers and professionals not to pathologise or judge chemsex. When they do, not only do they diminish an experience that can be both good and bad, but they also allow prejudice to potentially interfere with support for community members who need it, which can be disastrous.

For example, in 2016, a man named Stephen Port was convicted for the rape and murder of four men using GHB. According to the coroner's report, police errors – including a failure to link two victims found in the same position in the same graveyard and killed with the same drug – likely contributed to three of the deaths. In 2018, the Independent Office for Police Conduct investigated officers involved. Though the investigation found performance failings for nine officers, none were disciplined and five have since been promoted.[6] There are many similar examples of how prejudice towards LGBTQIA+ people leads police to ignore or mishandle violence towards them. Often, institutions outwardly declare themselves tolerant and inclusive while at the same time judging the behaviour of marginalised groups because they have a different moral code. It's common to feel like institutions are fine with LGBTQIA+ people as long as they act like straight people. To deviate from straightness is to invite prejudice, silencing, and violence.

Seeking risky, dangerous, or harmful sex

Sex that can be classed as 'risky' or 'dangerous' can include many things. As we've discussed, chemsex is, by its very nature, risky because it involves using cocktails of drugs and potential sexual contact with multiple strangers. Other behaviours can also be risky for survivors.

Men who have been sexually abused in childhood or early adolescence may feel that their only currency is their sexual availability to others. Others' desire for them directly corresponds to their sense of worth. This can look different depending on the survivor. For example, some men risk everything – marriage, children, jobs – to hire sex workers or seek out sexual encounters outside their monogamous relationship.

I've worked with individuals who, as underage teenagers, sought out cruising or cottaging spots (areas where people meet for anonymous sexual encounters), sometimes for money but often for validation. In some cases, this behaviour *can* be a form of revictimisation. While it may not feel like victimisation at the time, the power dynamics involved can make it abusive and potentially illegal. This can reinforce the belief for survivors that their worth is tied to being a sexual object, while also exposing them to physical danger. Not every teenager who engages in cruising will see it as revictimisation or abuse, even if they were under the legal age of consent. Some may later reflect on the experience with a sense of wrongness, while others may not view it as abuse, considering it something they needed at that point in their lives. Crucially, each individual's feelings and experiences are paramount in understanding and responding to these situations.

This is a complex issue, and I encourage survivors to be their own guide in determining whether they were revictimised, retraumatised, or made sexual decisions simply based on where they were and what they wanted at that time in their lives. For allies of survivors who have experienced this, I urge you to set aside your moral judgements and allow yourself to be guided by the survivor you are supporting, it is them who will tell you whether this experience, to them, was abusive or not.

In Chapter 4, we looked at the myth that men who were sexually abused go on to abuse others. This myth is untrue. However, as I explained in Chapter 4, a small number of male survivors do sexually harm others. They may do this through behaviours like public masturbation or flashing or more serious offences like assault. If a man commits sexual harm, it's unlikely to be because of an experience of sexual abuse alone. Rather, a combination of (often very tragic) events in his early life likely led him to seek control over others in this way. Again, this is not a result of his surviving sexual abuse alone but has to do with many complex variables or life events going wrong. Experiencing sexual abuse does not make a person sexually dangerous.

Some survivors may find themselves in extremely complex relationships with other people who have survived abuse. This dynamic can cause problems in situations where both partners are vulnerable in some way and one partner is easily influenced by uneven power dynamics. Consenting to sex can become complicated, particularly when practising BDSM or violent role play, in cases where consent is never discussed properly, or where one partner agrees to sexual acts they feel uncomfortable with because they don't want to disappoint or lose the other. These relationships can become codependent and enmeshed, and the lines between abuser and abused can be blurred.

Despite these complicated situations, on the whole, male survivors of sexual abuse are not a threat. On the contrary, men who survive abuse are more likely to do everything in their power to not be threatening, from avoiding walking behind women who are alone in the street to becoming celibate. Many male survivors can be so preoccupied with not being abusive that they develop anxiety about making others feel uncomfortable or scared.

A split between sex and intimacy

It's common for survivors to experience a split between their abilities to have sex and feel intimate. For example, a man may feel intense love and care for their partner but no feelings of eroticism. Try as they might, they are unable to feel sexual attraction towards the one person they are expected to feel sexual toward. The man may feel sexually attracted to others around them, possibly leading them to have emotionless sex outside their relationship. Or they might remember the passionate sex they had in the early days of dating their partner or the sex they had before the relationship and desperately want to return to it. For many survivors who face it, this is a painful experience. It is another example of how sex can create a double life, one part sexless and difficult, the other part dark, sex-driven, and shameful. These difficult feelings can become much worse if our partner blames themselves for not being attractive or if they accuse us of not being strong and manly enough to have sex with them.

Some survivors cultivate relationships with people who, for their own reasons, also don't act on their sexual desires. These sexless relationships can be affectionate, full of touch and emotional closeness. While these relationships may be ideal most of the time, a lack of sex can feel like a taboo that neither partner wants to talk about for fear of the damage it may cause. Such relationships may be monogamous or ethically non-monogamous, in which each partner might have sex with other people. Counterintuitively, consensual sex outside the relationship can make the lack of sex in the relationship feel even more difficult. Sometimes, partners in these non-sexual relationships seek out threesomes or group sex. While this may sound exciting and liberating, it can be a way of avoiding one-to-one sex on an intimate, romantic level. Group sex soon becomes frustrating, as one or both partners miss the authentic emotional connection that came from being together.

Disconnecting from sex

In a room of male survivors, it's common to find that a percentage of them have no interest in sex or relationships. It's important not to confuse these men with aromantic or asexual people, who have little or no interest in sexual or romantic attraction. Survivors who remain abstinent may feel sexually attracted to others or wish for a relationship but be overwhelmed by the idea of seeking one out. They may feel that 'the ship has sailed' and they have missed the chance to find a partner. Often, they bury any sexual desire, simply not allowing it to feature in their daily life. Some survivors may feel intense anxiety or fear around the idea of sexual relationships or connections. The phenomenon of losing the appetite for sex has been called *sexual anorexia*.

Survivors may feel a variety of ways about being disconnected from their Sexual Self. Some will feel sadness or frustration that they are unable to pursue sexual relationships, while others will be content not dating or having sex. This can depend on the individual's circumstances, how well they are able to support themselves and what access they have to society and friends.

Avoiding sex in relationships

For some men it is simply too difficult to know where to start when it comes to having sex. They are able to maintain loving relationships and might even sustain a sexual relationship with a partner for a short time, but eventually, the sex stops, and it becomes easier to avoid it altogether. To do this, men may use several tactics:

- Retreat into being a 'generous' lover, always willing to give partners sexual attention but never feeling safe enough to act on their own desires, even if partners give them permission or ask them to; this can slowly kill off any sexual spark in a relationship
- Avoid instigating sex altogether, feigning tiredness, illness or even starting a fight; some couples will throw themselves into a TV series and stay cuddling on the sofa until it's time to sleep; cuddling can be the death of eroticism
- Try to squash their partner's sex drive by blaming or punishing them for having sexual desires; 'You know I have work tomorrow'; 'I don't want to have sex; I have a lot on my mind'; or 'You're a sex addict'

Trauma responses to sex

Some men may desperately want to find partners, either romantic or sexual. They might be able to flirt in person or online, appearing to be sexually confident and experienced. However, there always comes a moment when trauma takes over. For example, a man may be talking in public with a potential sexual partner, only to freeze or feel compelled to flee the situation immediately. Other men find themselves starting sex with a partner, only for trauma to prevent it going any further. This can occur in various ways. Some men struggle to get or maintain an erection, while others may suddenly have a flashback to a traumatic event. Still others may feel their confidence escape and worry about assaulting the person they are with, rather than staying in the moment and letting their Sexual Self be free with the other person. Some men consider sexual prowess a key part of what makes them a man. Not being able to perform in the way they want or having a profound trauma response in the build-up to or during sex can feel shameful. There is an assumption that if men are not having sex or find sex complicated, there is something wrong with them. This creates a lonely and shameful mindset that is hard for many to escape.

Some survivors may encounter *traumatic loneliness*, which occurs when the impact of sexual abuse is so profound that it's impossible for the survivor to find any intimacy with other people. Traumatic loneliness looks different for different people. Some men form addictions or compulsive needs that help numb the traumatic pain. These needs can become acute and eclipse all other relationships as the survivor prioritises the addiction over friends or family. Other men may find any contact at all with people to be too much. They assume the worst of people and feel like no one will ever understand. Even when loved ones try to reach out, they find ways to jeopardise the connection early to avoid disappointment later.

Difficulty accepting the experience of sexual abuse

It may be difficult for some survivors to accept they were sexually abused in the first place. This can happen under many circumstances. For example, if a man is coerced or peer-pressured into having sex, particularly with a woman, they might not even recognise the experience as abuse. Feelings of discomfort and powerlessness are repressed or explained away as chaotic or due to inexperience, particularly if the abuse happened when they were teens or young adults. Men are often rewarded with high social status or told they are lucky for being sexually active. In this environment, it can feel inappropriate for men to classify unwanted sex as abuse. However, as survivors think back, the discomfort often grows, causing any number of challenging sexual behaviours, from sexual anorexia to compulsively seeking sex to feel in control.

7.3 Society vs identity, gender, and sexual preference

Male survivors often face multiple myths and stigma that can be easy to internalise. Some men face myths and stigma about their sex and gender identity on top of the stigma they endure from the sexual abuse. Societal views on these men's sexual identity can affect the quality of support they are able to receive as survivors. This is an intersectional issue, as some men not only live with a seldom-talked-about trauma but also battle prejudice, stereotype, or fetishisation.

Black men, for example, are often fetishised and stereotyped as overly masculine, hypersexual, and promiscuous. This practice is degrading, defining Black men around the sexual desires or racist beliefs of others. It is particularly dangerous to Black male survivors for several reasons. Black men may face additional bigotry when accessing either support or justice systems. This plays out an oppressive argument with a long history: that Black people are biologically different from white people, positioning them as 'other' – more hypersexualised, more masculine, more promiscuous, etc. This assertion has been used as justification for policing and controlling Black people for decades, and its consequences live on today. Often, when a Black survivor decides to report or seek help for sexual abuse or rape they have experienced, they cannot be certain that the colour of their skin will not affect the quality of support they get from police and the healthcare and criminal justice systems.

Autistic men can also have their sexual identities stereotyped. Often, autistic men are seen as sexually childlike – disinterested or incapable of intimate romantic relationships. Not only is good representation absent, but a much larger problem exists. According to the Autism Research Institute, 'a lack of personal and clinical education combined with communication and social differences leaves many autistic people prone to abuse'.[7] Further, the institute notes, autistic young people are three to four times more likely to experience sexual victimisation than non-autistic young people. Because society denies autistic men a Sexual Self, it also denies them space to talk about intimate relationships and discuss consent and healthy versus unhealthy relationships. This impacts autistic men's ability to report abuse or rape.

The support trans and transmasculine people who survive abuse are able to access is limited. Although trans people occupy an extremely small percentage of the population, they are disproportionally affected by gender violence. While campaigning and support is sparsely available, it is often focused on support for trans women. It is rare to find help or research geared specifically towards transmasculine people's experience of sexual abuse. FORGE, a US charity that works with transgender communities, conducted one such study in 2011, using 1,005 participants and found that transmasculine people were more likely to be victims of childhood and adult sexual abuse, domestic violence, and stalking.[8]

Even when support services are available to trans men, staff rarely have the expertise required to understand these survivors' experience. This leaves many trans men in the UK to navigate the complicated landscape of rape and sexual abuse services by themselves. Making it harder, some of these services have been pulled into the problematic debates about gender-critical versus gender-affirming beliefs. A trans man might find a service with a short therapy waiting list, sexual trauma skills, and a low or free cost that may dispute his gender or refuse to work with him. This isolates survivors or forces them to hide parts of their identity, while also shutting down any essential conversations survivors may want to have about gender and identity. I once spoke with the service manager of a well-known male sexual abuse service who told me that a large number of self-referrals to the service listed their gender as male *and* gender questioning. Importantly, this tells us *not* that sexual abuse makes people trans, but that it is such a powerful trauma that it often affects all parts of us. As men work to recover from this painful and confusing experience, they must examine many parts of themselves that those who have not experienced abuse seldom have to navigate (more on this in Chapter 4, 'Masculinity'). Charities that do not work with trans men may shut down conversations that many cisgender men, whose gender identity aligns with their gender assigned at birth, may want to have about gender.

It is not just survivors' identity that can fall victim to stereotypes and prejudice, but their sexual preferences too. Few sexual practices are as misunderstood or stigmatised as kink. I've sat with countless people of all genders who have felt shamed or judged for desiring kinky sex. For survivors, this shame can be especially acute, as many wrongly associate kink with childhood sexual abuse. In truth, curiosity about kink develops either internally during childhood or much later, in adulthood. Many people interested in kink remember watching a TV show or films in which a character was tied up and could not move, as in the heroine tied to the train tracks in old Western films or the cartoon hero strapped to a chair for interrogation. For some children, these scenes are transfixing. Importantly, they are not sexual as adults think of it, but they do mark the start of a curiosity about power, being held and submission. In adulthood, interest in kink may come through exposure to pornography or kinky partners who act as a gateway.

Some survivors interested in kink do recreate, in role play, the sexual abuse they survived. This can be confusing for the survivor. If they enjoy the role play, they think, surely a part of them enjoyed the abuse as well. In my experience, this is not the case. More likely, survivors use kinky role play to relive an experience where they were powerless and unable to consent, this time giving themselves agency. This time, they are strong and consenting. They are taking power back and alleviating trauma through play. This is counter to the common misconception that sexual trauma is the cause of kink; rather, kink is a tool used to detraumatise the abuse. It's worth noting that the results of this play are often mixed. While I've worked with some survivors for whom recreating abuse helped, for others it was very difficult and confusing. Whatever the result, it is worth remembering that the behaviour is driven by a desire to feel better, rather than a secret enjoyment of the abuse.

From an intersectional perspective, kink communities tend to be more inclusive than other adult spaces, such as bars, pubs, straight sex parties, or clubs. Generally, there is greater acceptance in kink communities of people from minority backgrounds, as well as people with different body types, disabilities, genders, and sexualities. As we've seen in throughout this book, trauma and abuse tend to be more pervasive in minoritised communities. It seems possible that the kink community has a higher awareness of trauma and the importance of reaching a firm agreement on boundaries and consent. Again, this is the opposite to stereotypes that suggest kink is simply violent, uncaring, and retraumatising sex. These stereotypes ignore or are unaware of consent practices common in kink communities, including safe words (words to stop sexual activities when they become uncomfortable), traffic light systems ('red', 'amber', and 'green', which indicate stopping, pausing, and starting or continuing sexual activities) and after care, (post-sex re-centring, such as cuddling, talking about the sex, rehydrating, and caring for each other). Of course, kinky spaces can still carry risk. Engaging in extreme practices can be retraumatising, and there are plenty accounts of abuse in kink spaces. However, the same can be said of nightclubs and bars everywhere. What is important here is that whatever your sexual choices and likes, you know that they are *yours*. Conflating them with sexual abuse is simplistic at best and harmful at worst.

Every person faces many potential barriers to discovering their Sexual Self. Add the experience of sexual abuse, stereotypes and issues around identity, and it's easy to see why many male survivors keep their Sexual Self hidden from the world. After all, a hidden Sexual Self is harder to abuse and retraumatise. However, while hiding our Sexual Self may protect it for a while, it also stops us from healing and growing. Finding ways to be comfortable with our Sexual Self can take time. It's been with us since we were very young, so treating it in a kind, childlike way can be a useful start. Give yourself permission to be curious about yourself and what you do and don't like. In the next chapter, we will discuss trust and how to develop it. Perhaps applying some of the tools we discuss there will help you connect with who you are sexually, whatever that means for you as an individual. I want to leave this chapter with a quote from American writer Augusten Burroughs' book *Possible Side Effects*: 'Sexual Self-discovery is not just about pleasure; it's about learning who you are and what you want, and having the confidence to go after it'.[9]

Letter Writing

Letter writing can be a powerful way to connect with our emotions. Many survivors find that writing a letter to their past self, offering forgiveness, can help reduce feelings of shame. Others write to their future self, offering hope. Some choose to write letters to people, both living and deceased, who have played significant roles in their lives. There are even those who write to their perpetrator, expressing how the sexual abuse has affected them.

These letters are rarely sent. Instead, they are often kept, burned, or filed away. The purpose isn't to deliver the message but to express your feelings and say what you need to say. If you're considering writing a letter, I suggest starting with one to yourself, either to your past or future self. This can be surprisingly emotional, so it's often helpful to begin with yourself before addressing a parent, caregiver, or perpetrator, especially if your feelings toward them are complex.

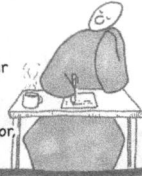

Dear...

For A4 and printable versions of this worksheet, visit www.jeremysachs.com

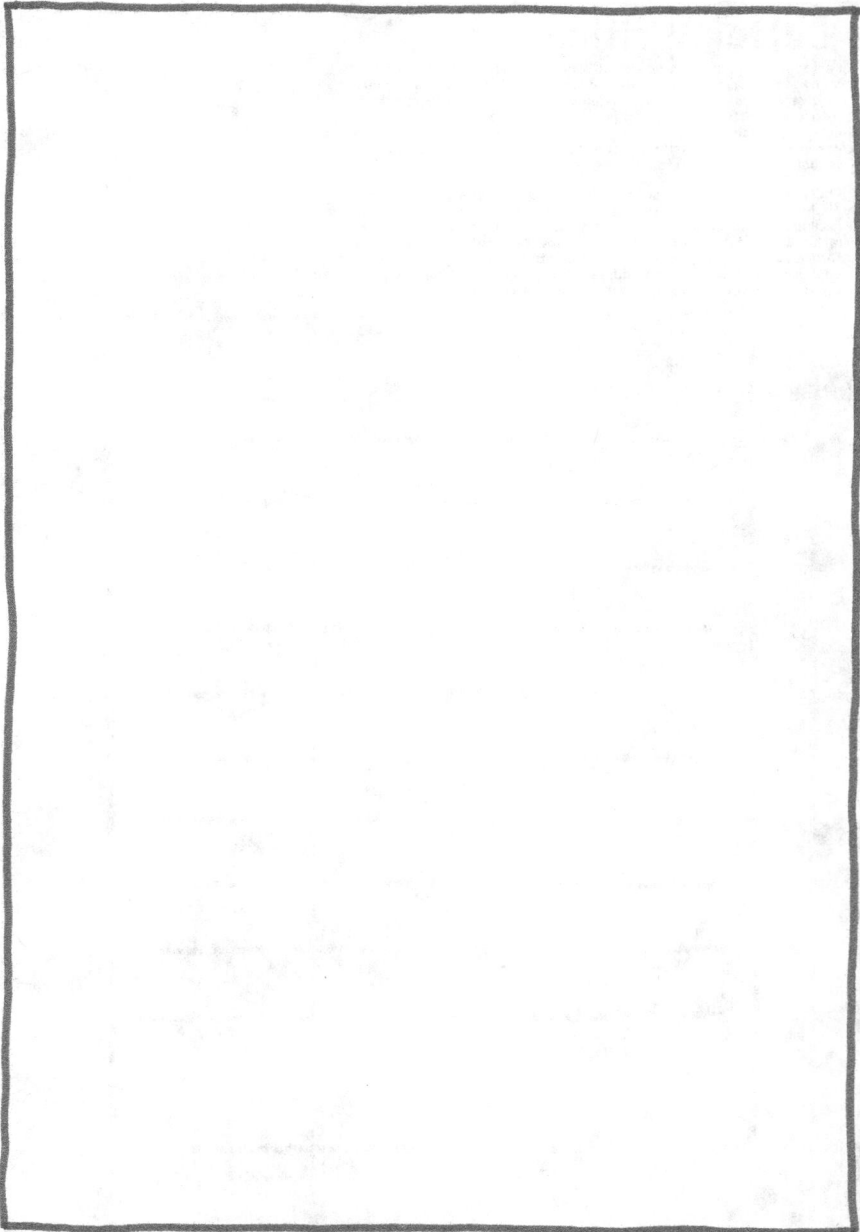

www.jeremysachs.com   @JeremySachs_

For A4 and printable versions of this worksheet, visit www.jeremysachs.com

Resources

The Trauma Talks podcast, series 1, episode 5: 'Chemsex' by Jeremy Sachs and Katherine Cox

My podcast explores a different experience of trauma in each episode. This episode speaks to people who have survived sexual abuse and used chemsex.

BDSM and Kink: The Basics *by Stefani Goerlich and Elyssa Helfer*

ISBN 9781032320632
This book takes a sex-positive, kink-affirming approach to the material, exploring everything from basic terminology to risk assessment and clinical best practices.

I May Destroy You (2020)

This limited TV series was created by Michaela Coel with a predominantly Black British cast. It follows Arabella, a young writer, as she rebuilds her life after being raped. The series also includes a storyline featuring Kwame, a Black British gay man and friend of Arabella, who is raped during a Grindr meet-up.

Signposting

Fumble

https://fumble.org.uk
This is an award-winning youth charity in the UK, leading the way in supporting young people with their mental and sexual health and relationships in the digital age.

Terrence Higgins Trust

www.tht.org.uk
This is one of the leading sexual health charities in the UK, focusing on HIV and sexual health education, prevention and support services.

Sex Positivity UK

www.sexpositivityuk.com
Resources and a psychosexual therapist directory created by Silva Neves, one of the critical friends who offered feedback on this chapter. The website promotes a sex-positive, science-led, evidence-based approach to compulsive sexual behaviours.

Notes

1 Avodah Offit, *The Sexual Self: How Character Shapes Sexual Experience* (New York: Meridian, 1983).
2 World Health Organization, 'Compulsive sexual behaviour disorder', in *International Classification of Diseases*, 11th Revision (ICD-11) (Geneva: World Health Organization, 2019).
3 Johannes Fuss, Jared W. Keely, Dan J. Stein, Tahilia J. Rebello, José Ángel García, Peer Briken, et al., 'Mental health professionals' use of the ICD-11 classification of impulse control disorders and behavioral addictions: An international field study', *Journal of Behavioral Addictions* (12 January 2024): 276–292, https://doi.org/10.1556/2006.2023.00083.
4 'International Classification of Diseases 11th Revision (ICD-11) for Mortality and Morbidity Statistics', World Health Organization, 2024. https://icd.who.int/browse/2024-01/mms/en#1630268048, accessed 30 July 2024.
5 'Chemsex', *The Trauma Talks*, series 1, episode 5 (Apple Podcasts, 6 October 2020), https://podcasts.apple.com/gb/podcast/1-5-the-trauma-talks-chemsex/id1517405491?i=1000493838207, accessed 2 August 2024.
6 'Inspection of the Metropolitan Police Service's response to lessons from the Stephen Port murders', Her Majesty's Inspectorate of Constabulary and Fire & Rescue Services (HMICFRS), 27 April 2023. https://hmicfrs.justiceinspectorates.gov.uk/publication-html/inspection-of-the-metropolitan-police-services-response-to-lessons-from-the-stephen-port-murders, accessed 2 August 2024.
7 'Sexual victimization in autism', Autism Research Institute, 2024. https://autism.org/sexual-victimization-in-autism/#:~:text=Autistic%20youth%20are%20three%20to,Weiss%20%26%20Fardella%2C%202018, accessed 2 August 2024.
8 Loree Cook-Daniels, 'Op-ed: trans men experience far more violence than most people assume', *The Advocate*, 23 July 2015, https://www.advocate.com/commentary/2015/07/23/op-ed-trans-men-experience-far-more-violence-most-people-assume, accessed 5 August 2024.
9 Augusten Burroughs, *Possible Side Effects* (New York: St. Martin's Press: 2006).

Chapter 8

Trust and the bitter legacy of betrayal

Chapter Contents

Trust and identity

As a trans man who survived sexual abuse, trust is something I've had to work really hard to understand and rebuild. When I was younger, before I knew I was trans, I was sexually abused. My mum would drop me off at a private tutor's house and he'd show me pornography as if it was all part of the tutoring. He'd ask me if I wanted to be touched or whether I'd want to touch myself like in the pornography. I think I already had dysphoric feelings towards my body and my genitals at that age, but seeing the pornography made me feel numb towards my body. I don't know if that's how I felt then, or this is me looking back on it. This went on for a year. By then, I became really angry and was sent to see a counsellor, who also abused me. It only happened once, as I was older and didn't have to go back. What stays with me now is how smug the counsellor was. They didn't try and hide anything, like they just knew they could get away with it, like they took one look at me and felt like they could do whatever they wanted to me. They could see I was vulnerable and did it anyway, or even because I was vulnerable. It messed me up in a lot of ways, making me feel like I couldn't trust anyone, including myself. I felt completely disconnected from my own body and my sense of self. I think it probably delayed me coming out as trans for years because of all the confusion the abuse caused.

Coming out to my family was a huge relief, but I still didn't tell people about the abuse. I still mix them up in my head even though I know the abuse has nothing to do with my gender. It's hard to separate them. It's like a bowl of spaghetti trying to detangle different strands in my head but

DOI: 10.4324/9781003423331-8

it's all jumbled up. On top of that, people assume trans people have been abused or that they are somehow dangerous or sexually manipulative. It's hard not to internalise all that, like, did I lead on my tutor and counsellor? This makes it hard to trust myself and I can really feel worthless. Then trusting others becomes hard when they might reject you or even be violent towards you.

I lost friends and some family members when I transitioned. But I was lucky to have supportive close family and friends. Even if I couldn't talk about the abuse, talking about my gender was helpful. Some people were difficult at first, but they came around and, to their credit, educated themselves, which helped. I learned that trust isn't about expecting perfection, but about finding people who respect me. Once I was out, things started to feel better, like at least one part of me was living authentically.

One of the toughest parts was learning to trust my own feelings and instincts again. I spent so long doubting myself and my worth. I started by setting small boundaries and listening to what I needed. Every time I respected my own boundaries, I felt a little more confident in myself.

Now, I see trust as something that can grow and change over time. It's not all-or-nothing (which is a huge change from when I was younger). I've learned to trust in my own ability to heal. For me, the next step is working out how to talk about the abuse without sending me back to a dark place or ruining my family. It feels like it never ends, but I'm in a better place now than before because I can trust myself.

Bex, transgender man (he/him/they/them), disabled, 32 years old

Trust can feel abstract when we try to pin down what it actually is. We can go weeks not thinking about trust until a situation arises where we need it. We might learn a secret or need advice about a sensitive situation. Then we search our minds for people we can trust. And if trust is broken, the emotional fallout can be so all-consuming that we become suspicious of future friendships or relationships.

This is why, in my groups, we create a working definition of trust, which goes along the following lines: Trust is the feeling of being able to put down the protective shield men wear around our vulnerabilities. Not everyone can be trusted 100 per cent, so some men only put that protective shield down partially. Each new person requires an assessment of trustworthiness and the amount of protective shielding we need to keep on or take off. This can change over time. Some people may feel completely trustworthy, like our trust in them is made of concrete. Other people may require constant work, as we might trust them with some things, but not others. All of my groups seem to agree that once trust has been broken, it can be hard to get it back, especially for survivors.

8.1   Trust

Not everyone feels the need to consciously think about trust. Some people effort-lessly trust the safety of their environment and rarely feel endangered. Even if they do occasionally sense danger, they trust the world to correct any wrongs they experience. They trust friends to back them up in arguments and services like law enforcement or healthcare organisations to act in their best interest. In an ideal world, I'd argue trust begets trust: the more we are able to trust, the more trust we will receive back.

We need trust so much that our entire species depends on it. It's been an evolu-tionary imperative for millennia: we share knowledge, form bonds, start families, and distribute resources. Despite being necessary since the beginning of our spe-cies, trust is not a static thing. We're constantly making up our minds about people's trustworthiness. It's fluid and changeable depending on how a person or situation makes us feel. As Peter A Hancock and colleagues wrote in 2011, we 'learn to calculate exposure to the risk of harm from the actions of an influential other'.[1] In other words, we learn to assess the potential risk of physical or psychological harm from others and decide how much to trust them based on our assessment. However, for a survivor, trust can be especially difficult. Having our trust broken by sexual abuse can feel like a wound that never properly heals. Each new betrayal of trust, from bad relationships to social inequalities, risks further wounding.

To understand how important trust is and how easily it can be wounded, it helps to look at where trust originates. Trust starts early. From the moment we are born, it's crucial that we trust those around us. As infants, we don't understand the con-cept of trust in the same way adults, but we are still beginning to trust. We trust we'll be fed when hungry, picked up when scared, and given a blanket when cold. This early sense of trust is cumulative; if a parent fed an infant yesterday and feeds them today, the infant will learn to trust they'll be fed tomorrow as well. Small les-sons like this are essential to the growing infant and allow them to trust the world is safe.

One scholar who thought a lot about trust in infancy is Erik Erikson. Erikson was a German Jewish psychologist born in 1902. He grew up with a sense that he was different. His mother, Karla Abrahamsen, was Jewish, and his father's identity was never revealed, although it was guessed that he was a non-Jewish tourist from Denmark. Erikson grew up being bullied for looking Nordic, while non-Jewish children subjected him to antisemitism. This perhaps had an impact on his work as it concerned how social experiences shape people.

Erikson worked to understand the impact of social experiences on people as they age, and he devised a model for the stages of psychosocial development. The first stage, which occurs between birth and 18 months, is the development of trust versus mistrust. Erikson asserted that infants are born anxious about the world and rely on their parent or primary caregiver for constant, stable care. If the par-ent or primary caregiver is reliable, nurturing, and consistent, the infant stands a good chance of developing a sense of trust. The infant *trusts* the world is safe and people around them are reliable; the parent who fed them yesterday and today will also feed them tomorrow. This becomes the infant's baseline trust level, so even if something threatening happens, they return to this safe and trusting way of being. Erikson believed that infants who psychologically survive this stage will trust those around them to meet their needs and support them even if bad things happen. These infants develop what he called 'the virtue of hope'.[2] Erikson believed that this virtue was essential for developing trust and healthy relationships. He wrote, 'Hope is both the earliest and the most indispensable virtue inherent in the state of being alive. If life is to be sustained hope must remain, even where confidence is wounded, trust impaired'.[3] Correspondingly, Erikson argued that infants who receive inconsistent or inadequate care from those around them will fail to develop the virtue of hope and instead develop fear – a sense that relationships around them cannot be trusted. This infant may grow up experiencing low self-esteem, anxiety, or mistrust, unable to believe that they have worth or can influence the world around them.

We also know that infants who experience unstable starts in life can be at greater risk of sexual abuse. For example, the 2023 Australian Child Maltreatment Study found that young people in institutional care have a higher lifetime prevalence of sexual victimisation compared to the rest of the population.[4] A 2017 German study published in *Child Abuse and Neglect* found that boys in residential care or boarding schools were 8 per cent more likely to experience sexual abuse.[5] This suggests that certain circumstances, such as the environment we are raised in and our parents' ability to meet our needs, can combine with sexual abuse to create a potent mix of experiences that prevent us trusting others.

Of course, you might also be reading this thinking, *My childhood was good. This doesn't apply to me, but it's still difficult to trust people. Why!?* It's possible that you struggle with trust because it isn't a skill we ever fully master. No one gets to adulthood knowing exactly how to do it. We all remain vulnerable to breaches of trust. Some breaches are so drastic that they can destabilise our mental health from any point in our life onwards. Sexual abuse is one such breach. Abuse can be an experience that feels like it changes everything. We may go from being someone who is able to trust the world to someone who sees danger everywhere. The power of sexual abuse and the damage it causes can be an ultimate betrayal.

8.2   Betrayal

When we define *betrayal* in my groups, there are common elements most survivors agree on. Betrayal feels like a deliberate and proactive choice that is directly harmful to a person or group. It is especially wounding because a betrayal doesn't simply do harm but also leaves us with a sense of being failed. A parent who abuses a child not only harms them but also fails to protect them as a parent should. This breaks the expectation of trust – the social contract that a parent should protect their child. If a friend betrays us by lying, it is not just the lie that hurts but the realisation that someone we thought was trustworthy is not.

As children, we live in a social contract with our parents: the child loves the parent unconditionally, and in return, the parent takes care of and loves the child. Inevitably, somewhere during the child's development, the parent breaks the social contract, leaving the child feeling betrayed. This betrayal may be an everyday mistake or a conflict of interest:

- Missing sports games or performances
- Not buying the correct birthday present
- Forbidding friendships or social activities
- Failing to protect the child from minor disappointments
- Severely scolding the child
- Prioritising work or other commitments before the child's needs

Betrayals like these happen every day, to (I suspect) everyone. While they may be difficult for children, they're probably not abuse or neglect, and though we may want to protect children from such betrayal, the experience can be useful. If children's virtue of hope remains intact, they can feel betrayed by a parent and, because they also feel love from the same parent, return to safety. The child hopefully learns that betrayal is survivable and relationships can be repaired. This is a useful lesson for use following future betrayals.

Of course, some children experience much more damaging betrayals that turn their life upside-down. The betrayal is too emotionally powerful for them to recover from it. Betrayal can stay with the child long into adulthood, including having parents or close adults who

- Rely on alcohol or drugs and cannot fully connect with the child
- Have depression and struggle to emotionally meet the child's needs or make them feel seen
- Are abusive towards another family member in the child's presence
- Are abusive towards the child in any way, including physically, sexually, emotionally, or neglectfully
- Are inconsistent, sometimes offering the child what they need and sometimes being absent, abusive, scary or indifferent
- Have a child who needs to be taken into care by local authorities
- Die or leave the child or family

Sexual abuse is a betrayal of the law, social and familial norms, and our right to autonomy. It can feel like a betrayal no matter what age we were when we experienced it, and this feeling may worsen, depending on whether the people around us help us find our virtue of hope or further betray us. Survivors may seek a restorative experience through legal proceedings that can further betray us because the legal system is disjointed and unbalanced in its convictions. As Dame Vera Baird, the Victims' Commissioner for England and Wales wrote in her *2021/22 Annual Report*,

> For victims, reporting rape is effectively a lottery and the odds are rarely in your favour. In the year to December 2021, there were 67,125 rape offences recorded – an all-time high. Yet the number of completed rape prosecutions plummeted from 5,190 in 2016/17 to just 2,409 in 2020/21. The numbers of convictions almost halved (2,689 in 2016/17 compared to 1,409 in 2020/21). Only 5 per cent of rapes that were given an outcome by the police in the year ending December 2021 resulted in a charge.[6]

In the following sections, I have categorised betrayal into three different types: betrayal by *people*, *organisations*, and *ourselves*. Hopefully, you'll find some of your experiences represented here. However, betrayal is so personal to each individual. If you don't find an example close to your experience, you may want to try using the blank page at the end of this chapter to write, doodle, draw, or process the ways you feel betrayed.

Betrayal by people

Incest/family

The very word *incest* has the power to be deeply upsetting. The experience itself can be psychologically devastating and have lifelong consequences as the abused child grows into adulthood. I have seen clients in their seventies who came to therapy for the first time for support working through sexual abuse by a family member over a half century earlier. This trauma's longevity may be in part because the relationship between the survivor and perpetrator has been enmeshed in a cycle of abuse, power, and need, often over many years. Abuse by a family member responsible for your care can confuse and shatter trust. While the word *incest* describes sexual abuse perpetrated specifically by a biological relative, the impact of abuse by an older person with similar power and trust – like a family friend, foster carer, or step-parent – can be equally harmful.

Often, incest can become complicated, involving more people than just survivor and abuser. Even if there is only one perpetrator in the family, certain conditions within the family may exist that allow the abuse to take place. Chaotic or abusive household environments can mean sexual abuse goes unnoticed. In some cases, family members may be so emotionally repressed or the family dynamics so dysfunctional that members ignore or deny that suspected abuse is happening. When this happens, the break in trust occurs between the survivor and their whole family on many different levels.

Incest can provoke a particular type of shame for survivors. We may feel entirely responsible, left with a dark secret that we cannot tell anyone, even our own family.

The topic of incest occupies positions in Western society that seem opposed to each other. In most public settings, it is considered unthinkable and deeply wrong. Yet, according to Bedbible, 50 per cent of videos on the pornography website PornHub are incestuous in nature, and the quantity of these videos grew an average of 1.5 per cent each year between 2015 and 2022.[7] Some speculate that this is due to TV shows like *Game of Thrones* and *House of the Dragon*, which feature incest plot lines. References to incest in popular culture can be deeply troubling for survivors and may represent a break in trust between us and the rest of society. They can leave survivors feeling on the outside, isolated, looking in at a society that doesn't understand or care about our experience.

Responsible adults

Outside the family, children come into contact with countless adults who are responsible for their growth and development, as well as their safety. Youth workers, bus drivers, babysitters, au pairs, sports coaches, arts and drama teachers (the list could go on endlessly) all hold positions of power and responsibility. Children and teenagers trust these people inherently because society tells them that they should. Sexual abuse by a responsible adult is distressing and confusing because, as children, we are told to behave and do as adults tell us to do. Children are often given messages like, 'Be good at school and listen to your teacher', or 'Music lessons are expensive, so work hard'.

On top of this, some children and teenagers are particularly vulnerable to abuse by predatory adults who come into contact with them. Often, abusive adults target young people who are already marginalised in some way, as they may be easier to isolate and groom. This makes already vulnerable children even more vulnerable.

Friends

Though sexual abuse perpetrated by a friend can fall into most of these categories, it is also worth highlighting by itself because of how disturbing the experience can be. Sexual abuse betrays our trust, right to consent or have agency over ourselves, *and* previous positive memories and experiences with the perpetrator. It can also have unforeseen consequences, such as turning friendship groups in on each other, leaving survivors on the outside at our most vulnerable moment. The abuse not only robs the survivor of trust in the friendship but can also take away their entire support system.

Online networks, messaging boards, and social media

The online world moves fast. A growing number of people are experiencing abuse online. This can feel isolating, as support services, therapists, and the general discourse around online sexual abuse can feel out of date. I speak to many survivors who describe having to not only disclose their experiences to therapists but also act as educators on online chat platforms. Online abuse is not a new problem, but it is an ever-changing one. Online sexual abuse often involves some type of grooming or coercion luring the victim into an online sexual act, such as sharing sexual pictures, videos, or audio of themselves. The betrayal can come in a variety of forms, from perpetrators sharing nude photos publicly or on pornography websites or networks to lying about their identity in order to gain trust and exploit victims.

Dating apps

A 2023 scoping review published in the journal *Trauma, Violence, and Abuse* found that sexual harassment was highly prevalent in dating apps. In fact, the review found that across 12 studies, between 57 and 88.8 per cent of people had experienced harassment. Women and individuals who identified as members of a sexual minority group were at highest risk, and harassment either took place online or in person after meeting through the app.[8]

While sexual harassment is different from abuse, it can still be psychologically disturbing, especially if we have experienced abuse before. It can bring up bad memories from the past and compound feelings of aloneness and isolation. A study published in *The Journal of Sex Research* in 2023 highlighted how using dating apps can facilitate sexual violence among student populations, again, disproportionately impacting women and members of sexual minority groups.[9] This kind of betrayal can feel similar to that experienced by people who are abused online. However, dating app abuse differs because we meet people through apps and are lulled – through our hopes of a new relationship, fun night out or new experience – into a false sense of security or fondness, only to be sexually harassed or assaulted in person.

Betrayal by institutions

The religious, statutory and community institutions in our lives hold substantial power and influence. We expect them to look after us, keep us safe, build community, and support our healing and social growth and development. We often feel institutional betrayal as being twofold: we are first betrayed by an individual connected to the organisation and second by the organisation itself, which failed to protect us or support us after the abuse. The disparity of power between survivors and institutions is such that the abuse can be particularly isolating, leading us to feel outside and isolated from the institution. The following sections represent a few examples.

Religious

Religious organisations historically held – and, in many parts of the world, continue to hold – huge influence and power over communities. A religious leader has not just spiritual power, but real-world power. They are often considered the representative of their god and therefore carry great authority. In many cases, abuse by a religious leader is comparable to incest in its impact, as many religions have strong symbolic father/mother symbolism, and religious congregations can become an extension of family.

Life-changing harm may result when someone who is raised within a belief system is then abused by that belief system, either by a religious leader or community member and/or through the organisation or community covering up the abuse. Such abuse alienates the survivor from the spiritual support they have been raised to believe in and leaves them feeling abandoned and worthless and questioning themselves. The imbalance of power in this type of abuse can be enormous. The survivor may feel that abuse they experience at the hands of religious leaders and organisations is also the will of a faceless, all-powerful god. Many religions have conservative or repressive attitudes towards sex, which can make abuse even more confusing and shaming for survivors.

In 2021, the UK's Independent Inquiry into Child Sexual Abuse released the report 'Child protection in religious organisations and settings', which found that sexual abuse happens in most religious organisations. In other words, no one religion is particularly prone to child sexual abuse. The report also found that many religious organisations do not have child protection policies and that victim blaming was common. Some religious communities do not have the language or capacity to describe rape or abuse, let alone report it. The report found that male victims of religious abuse far outnumber female victims. Researchers noted that there was

> no requirement on the part of the police to collect statistics at a national level in England and Wales as to the number of convictions or allegations relating to child sexual abuse in religious organisations and settings. There is no way of knowing the true scale of such abuse. [10]

Education

Schools, colleges, and universities are key places where young people develop and become independent. These places are full of information and first-time experiences. Future friends are made, career paths are decided, and exposure to lifelong hobbies is experienced. However, a 2023 University of Greenwich study of 593 male and female adults' retrospective accounts of secondary school (11–16 years old) in the UK and Ireland found that many people experienced sexual harassment by teachers or staff, both in person and online. Of UK respondents, 27 per cent said they had experienced unwanted sexual attention, compared to 7 per cent of Irish respondents. Further, 18 per cent of UK respondents had experienced at least one type of online sexual harassment. The study quotes one respondent saying, 'A teacher who I did not have messaged me on Grindr during school, I blocked him'.[11]

It is generally difficult to find studies of survivors who experienced abuse or rape in an educational setting. An exception to this is boarding schools. One investigation into abuse in residential schools, including boarding schools, found that

> [p]upils in boarding schools are vulnerable to both sexual abuse by adults working at the school and harmful sexual behaviour from other children. This is due to the features of the boarding school environment which mean there are greater opportunities for abuse to take place. Some of these features leading to increased risk apply equally to day pupils at boarding schools.[12]

Through my experience running groups and working with survivors in private practice, I have seen the damage that abuse at the hands of teaching staff can have on a survivor's life. Being abused by someone who holds such power over you in the context of an educational institution that also enforces rules and codes of conduct can be highly damaging. The abuse can be frightening, as when a teacher uses their power to isolate a student and silence them, or it can involve grooming, as when a teacher makes a student feel special and gives them special attention they may be missing in other parts of their life, only to break that trust through sexual abuse.

Educational intuitions can also provide a setting for student-on-student sexual abuse. According to a survey of 4,500 students conducted by the UK campaign Revolt, which aims to platform the voices of students abused on university campuses, 26 per cent of male students reported experiencing sexual violence at university. The same survey notes that

> *10 per cent of respondents reported their experiences of sexual violence to either the university or the police. When asked why, 56 per cent of students were convinced it 'wasn't serious enough'. 35 per cent felt too ashamed. 29 per cent did not even know how to make a report to the university. Only 2 per cent of those experiencing sexual violence felt both able to report it to their university and were then satisfied with the process.*[13]

Healthcare

Healthcare professionals hold huge amounts of power over children, teens, adults, and older adults alike. Not only do they represent an authority in the room, but we seek them out when we are unwell. We look to them to soothe both our physical and mental pain. Abuse at the hands of healthcare professionals can feel especially harmful because it is counterintuitive; we expect them to care for people, and yet abuse does happen. In fact, multiple types of abuse, from neglect to physical and even financial abuse, are carried out in nursing homes, hospitals, dentists' surgeries, psychotherapy rooms, and on home visits.

Sexual abuse often happens when victims are already vulnerable. Those seeking professional help for the repercussions of abuse may be abused again by a healthcare worker, and those who are vulnerable due to age, illness, disability, or treatment method may be targets for sexual abuse. Because there is often an enormous power imbalance between healthcare professionals and patients and because patients see healthcare professionals when we are vulnerable and need their help, this type of abuse can be very damaging. It can also damage survivors' future relationship with healthcare services, stopping us from seeking help with our physical and mental health.

Military, psychiatric hospitals, and prisons

Many institutions have long-established rules and cultural traditions that are internally upheld through a structured power system that is allowed to flourish behind closed doors. They are often self-regulated, a law unto themselves, meaning abuses of power often go unreported or, when they are reported, go unresolved. Institutions from the military to psychiatric hospitals and prisons rely by their very nature on a top-down power structure. Individual rights to freedom and privacy are removed, and this inevitably creates an ideal environment for exploitation and abuse.

The issue of sexual abuse in these types of institutions has been heavily studied. In 2018, the UK Care Quality Commission published a study finding that 273 alleged sexual assaults occurring in psychiatric facilities had been reported to the NHS during a period of three months.[14] I suspect that many cases in these settings go largely ignored because mentally ill or developmentally disabled victims have low social status and their voices are less heard and valued in institutions and society in general. According to a 1995 report published in the *Archives of General Psychiatry*, fewer men experienced sexual abuse within the US military than women, but among those who did, 65 per cent developed PTSD symptoms, compared to 39 per cent who experienced combat-associated trauma.[15] A 2016 study in the journal *Stress and Health* suggests that these men experienced PTSD symptoms over longer periods of time than female survivors.[16] In California, 59 per cent of transgender people in prison report having been sexually assaulted in prison, compared to 4.4 per cent of cisgender people in prison.[17] Despite the abundance of data, these numbers go largely unspoken about outside discussions around justice. The voices of people convicted of crimes rarely hold social capital and are often made up of society's most vulnerable populations, including people from minority backgrounds and people with mental health issues.

Institutional betrayal can be completely silencing. Institutions are by nature authoritarian, rarely allowing space for questions or criticism. This can leave survivors powerless multiple times over: the sexual abuse removes our agency to consent to sexual contact and the institution removes our agency to speak out or seek justice, all while failing to protect us from abuse in the first place.

Betrayal within ourselves

Betrayal of our own gender

Regardless of how we view masculinity, sexual abuse can be painful. Some men, particularly those who were abused by a man, find it extremely difficult to talk to or make friends with other men. One survivor told me, 'In social situations, I find a woman to hide behind. I don't know how to be with men. I don't want to talk to them'. Abuse at the hands of another man can confuse and hurt our relationship with our own gender. Men may feel unpredictable and dangerous. Some survivors develop a fear of masculinity that prevents male relationships and disconnects us from how it feels to be a man. This can become a vicious spiral where our inability to be comfortable with other men makes us feel further from our sense of ourselves as men. In turn, this may keep us feeling isolated or alone.

Trans male survivors can have a particularly complex relationship with their gender, often internalising the untrue myth that they are trans because of abuse. In addition, it can be upsetting for trans survivors to physically transition to the same visible gender as their perpetrator. Some trans men have shared with me that, to them, the male body feels synonymous with sexual abuse and the patriarchal oppression that allows so much abuse to go on; yet, in transitioning, they are, in some ways, working to look or dress or gain acceptance as a member of this gender. This can feel uneasy and bring up lots of questions for trans survivors about gender, shifting power, and finding their place in society.

Betrayal by our bodies

Often in discussions of sexual abuse, there is no question that the experience is violent and disturbing. What is rarely mentioned are the feelings of sexual excitement that victims may experience during abuse. It can be incredibly hard to make sense of this. If your body became aroused and/or orgasmed, you may feel like your body betrayed your psychological experience of distress. Survivors can be left asking ourselves, *Did I actually want the sexual contact?* This can lead us to minimise our trauma, say it wasn't that bad or spend years unsure if the abuse was, indeed, abuse. In some cases, perpetrators groom or condition victims for sex or sexual contact. By creating a sexual or suggestive atmosphere over prolonged periods, perpetrators can convince potential victims that we are the ones seeking out sexual contact. Even when we know it is abuse, we may still find ourselves habitually finding people who will abuse us or seeking out abusive sexual contact with a particular abuser.

Survivors who experienced physical arousal or instigated sexual contact with their perpetrator often feel confused and isolated, like no one would understand. I have met survivors who never disclosed their abuse in over a decade of therapy. It is important that we remember our body, particularly in vulnerable parts like our genitals, has thousands of nerve endings that are designed to be sensitive and respond to stimulation. Becoming erect or wet, orgasming, and feeling pleasurable sensations are only evidence of physical stimulus, not enjoyment or consent. Further, seeking out sexual contact from an abuser is an indicator of their power over you, not your desire for them. It is worth remembering that sexual contact cannot be consensual if a person abuses significant power over you or is threatening.

Betrayal of our trauma reaction

In some cases, we may feel like our body betrayed us by freezing during an assault. Men often feel like we could have fought off an abuser or escaped if only our body had not frozen. This is true even when we were assaulted as children; we still blame ourselves for not fighting off our attacker. Although there are good reasons for our bodies to freeze (see Chapter 2, page 28), the response can make us feel like we have betrayed our own masculinity.

Betrayal of our own decision making

Following abuse, many survivors have self-blaming thoughts, such as, *I should not have...*

- Drunk too much/taken drugs
- Gone home with that person
- Flirted so much
- Dressed like that
- Gone to that place
- Ignored my gut instincts
- Just let it happen
- Turned left when I normally turn right

Feeling like we were betrayed by our own decision-making process is often part of self-blame. Even if we know someone has wronged us, we still feel partly responsible. People around us may tell us we were not responsible for the abuse, but in many cases, a part of us struggles to believe it.

How betrayal can feel

Betrayal can feel intense and changeable. One minute, it can feel explosive and fiery and the next, numb and cold. Here are some emotions betrayal can cause:

- Rage
- Resentment
- Loneliness
- Shame
- Desire for forgiveness

- Isolation
- Jealousy
- Self-hatred or self-loathing
- Disgust
- Pining or desire
- Emasculation
- Resentment
- Numbness
- Sleepiness
- Regret
- Depression and/or anxiety

This list includes some wildly different emotions, and this should give you an indication of the power of betrayal. It can create powerful and contrasting emotions within us. It can also become habitual. We can learn to expect, and even anticipate, betrayal by people in our lives. This can create problems when we try to form new relationships and friendships. Primed for betrayal, we may become suspicious, and when it happens, it reinforces our anger or isolation and moves us even further from being able to trust.

Our inability to trust can become a prison where we get stuck, always looking out for betrayal and jealously resenting others. To break out of this prison, it can be useful to think about how we interact with other people and what we need to feel safe enough to start trusting in our relationships. Learning a little about attachment styles can help do this.

8.3   Attachment styles and steps towards trust

Attachment styles have gained a lot of attention recently. Thanks to social media and the self-help industry, more people are talking about their own style of attachment and wondering about the attachment styles of those they are closest to. When it comes to redeveloping trust after sexual abuse, attachment styles theory can help us better understand ourselves and our trust level.

Attachment styles theory was pioneered by psychiatrists John Bowlby and Mary Ainsworth. *Attachment styles* broadly refers to the patterns of relationships that we learn as infants and how it affects us in adulthood. In other words, how we were treated in childhood affects our confidence level around other people in adulthood. Attachments, according to this theory, fall into two types: secure and insecure.

Secure

Those of us who experience parenting where our needs are consistently met are likely to develop a secure base from which we can trustingly explore relationships and the world. This doesn't mean bad things don't happen or that we don't have anxieties or bad days; rather, we recover from times of distress or bad relationships fairly steadily. In this way, secure attachment is a bit like Erikson's 'virtue of hope', discussed earlier in this chapter. This is referred to as a secure attachment style.

What it feels like

This attachment feels able to be happy in company and by themselves. You can identify how you feel and, when you need to, communicate it to others. While not immune to social anxiety or awkwardness, someone with this attachment style is able to rally and recover in order to interact with others in a manageable, and productive way.

Examples

- Might feel nervous meeting a group of new people but is able to overcome those nerves and enjoy themselves
- Is able to navigate relationships (be it sexual or friendships) with boundaries and doesn't feel disproportionately reliant or frightened of others

Insecure

Abuse and other ACEs (see Chapter 2, page 52) can jeopardise children's ability to attach securely. Under adverse or abusive circumstances, a person is likely to develop one of the following insecure attachment styles: ambivalent, avoidant, or disorganised. While these develop in childhood, a version of them may follow a person into adulthood. You may be able to relate to some of them.

Ambivalent

WHAT IT FEELS LIKE

This attachment style can feel intense. People with an ambivalent attachment style frequently need reassurance in relationships and find it hard to trust without validation or reassuring time with partners or friends. Attempts at validation or reassurance can look to outsiders like clingy or possessive behaviour.

EXAMPLES

- When a partner or close friend does not message back quickly enough, it can spark an urgent need for reassurance and contact or even provoke anger and a sense of betrayal.
- Vague or unclear behaviour in a partner or close friend, even when trivial, can create a mix of emotions and responses, from wanting them to clarify what they meant to pushing boundaries or punishing them.

Avoidant

WHAT IT FEELS LIKE

This attachment style can feel deeply uncomfortable in emotional or intimate relationships. Closeness or people seeking closeness can make us want to keep emotional space between ourselves and those people. We may also find ourselves struggling with trust or using self-deprecating humour to avoid authentic emotional connection.

EXAMPLES

• We might keep partners or friends at a safe distance by avoiding deep conversations or changing the subject if people ask questions that feel intrusive.
• Someone expressing a desire to be emotionally closer to us might cause a strong emotional response such as anger, repulsion, cringe, or numbing.

Disorganised

WHAT IT FEELS LIKE

This attachment style can feel inconsistent and confusing. We might feel desperate to be close to someone one minute and want to push them away the next minute. It can feel like living with two opposing needs, one that wants to draw people close and the other that can't stand being close to people and pushes them away.

EXAMPLES

• We might feel like we're on an emotional rollercoaster, one minute pursuing closeness, the next feeling threatened or suffocated by the same closeness. This might lead us to overanalyse other people's behaviour or find it hard to trust or feel comfortable in relationships.
• Friends may accuse us of not respecting boundaries as we try to connect with or feel close to them; they may also accuse us of being avoidant or dismissive of the relationship.

An insecure attachment style can feel like a prison, especially if we find ourselves mistrusting people over and over again or trapped in a series of disappointing, betraying or abusive relationships. We might avoid attachment altogether due to fear of betrayal. I find it useful to think of insecure attachment styles like a big jacket. At some point in our past, we needed the big jacket because we were exposed to heavy rain, chilling winds, snow, and ice. The storm was so bad that even when it ended, we didn't take the jacket off. We anticipated the bad weather would return, even in the warmest climates, and why wouldn't we? The jacket might have saved our life. The trouble is, when it's warm, the jacket becomes too hot – even dangerous, in its own way.

Like the jacket, we wear our attachment style every day because at one point, it was necessary. When our environment changes and we continue anticipating betrayal, or even seeking it out, this attachment style no longer helps us and can even be harmful. But like the jacket, our attachment style is something we wear, not who we are. Just as we can change our jacket for any number of other items of clothing, so can we change how we attach to others. The change must be deliberate; in order to trust again, we need to expose ourselves to new experiences. This is how our brains grow and attachment styles alter. Of course, this is easier said than done.

Reflective activity

I often frame the stages of trust using the so-called 'Five Cs': *connection, caution, consistency, courage,* and *commitment.* Lots of models demonstrate steps towards trusting relationships, but the five stages in this model are particularly useful to the survivors I work with. They are useful to consider when stepping into new friendships or relationships, with either individuals or groups, in the context of hobbies, sports clubs, community activities, or therapy. The main thing the Five Cs communicate is that trust does not have to develop all at once. You can gently take small steps towards trusting a person and take small steps away if you feel they might not be completely trustworthy. The Five Cs also show that it is not necessarily appropriate to go through all five steps with everyone. You will meet people who aren't 100 per cent trustworthy, and that's okay; they can still be a friend.

When thinking about making new connections in your life and deciding how to trust them, have a go at applying these Five Cs. Ask yourself which stage a new relationship is at, which stage you want it to be at, what you need to do to make that happen and what you need from the other person.

1) **Connection.** In this stage, you have an initial spark of interest in someone. Something about them feels attractive, and you want to know more. If you've spoken to them, you might have an instinctive reaction or feel an innate energy between you.

2) **Caution.** In this stage, you expose a little more of yourself to the other person and notice how they respond. Do they feel safe to you? Do they react to you in a positive way? This may mean sharing

a joke or personal detail we wouldn't tell everyone and watching how they react. Do they react appropriately? If someone has broken our trust in a way that isn't too stressful or traumatic, this is often the stage we return to.

3) **Consistency.** In this stage, we build more regular connections. We seek out opportunities to spend time together and deepen the relationship. We expose more of ourselves, still testing for safety but finding more ease and beginning to foster intimacy in the relationship.

4) **Courage.** In this stage, we take a new risk in the relationship. We may introduce a new partner to friends and family, book a holiday with a new friend, or go on a weekend trip with a hobby group or sports team. Doing this can feel risky. If it goes wrong, the sense of betrayal could feel destabilising, but the reward would be a deeper investment in a more trusting relationship.

5) **Commitment.** In this stage, we are able to make gestures that show trust. This may include financial gestures, such as borrowing or lending money, or emotional gestures, such as offering a shoulder to cry on. It could mean baking the other person a cake or buying them a fridge magnet from a day trip. At this stage, you communicate that you are thinking of them and don't feel shy about showing fondness and care.

Developing trust after sexual abuse takes effort. This is hard for survivors because we have suffered a betrayal that feels catastrophic perpetrated by someone with power over us. Naturally, our instinct is to never let that happen again. Still, it's important that we get out of our comfort zone and give it a go. We can take small steps, experiment with starting conversations or join a therapy group or hobby club. If your first interaction doesn't go well, that's okay. Take a deep breath and move on to the next opportunity.

Managing autistic fatigue and burnout

Fatigue and burnout can happen to anyone. For autistic individuals, these can be more likely due to the pressures of social situations and sensory overload. If you're experiencing fatigue or burnout, it's crucial to manage your energy levels.

The National Autistic Society tells us autistic people can experience increased meltdowns and sensory sensitivity, physical pain and headaches, and shutting down physically, including loss of speech when fatigued and burned out.

If you're a survivor of trauma, managing it can exacerbate or accelerate autistic fatigue or burnout. Try the following strategies to help manage this, and remember: if things get really tough, reach out to a friend, therapist, or healthcare professional.

Energy Accounting

Energy accounting helps you set limits on your energy to avoid burnout. Estimate how much daily or weekly activities drain or energise you. Then, plan and balance your activities to manage stress, ensuring you include time for relaxation and recovery.

Time Off

Whether you use energy accounting or not, taking time off from work, school, and other high-stress activities is crucial for managing stress. Make sure to prioritise activities and interests that re-energise you and promote relaxation.

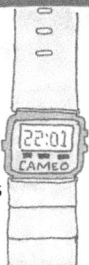

Time without Masking

Autistic people often feel the need to mask their traits in public, such as suppressing stimming, making eye contact, or mimicking social behaviours to fit in. This constant effort can be exhausting and contribute to fatigue. It's important to carve out times in your day where you are not masking, allowing yourself a safe and comfortable space.

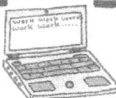

Manage Workload

To manage stress at work, track your workload and inform your manager if it becomes too much. Take regular breaks throughout the day to reset and ensure you plan and take your annual leave to recharge. Prioritising these strategies can help maintain a healthier work-life balance.

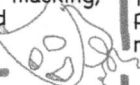

Manage Expectations

The pressure to meet expectations from employers, family, or friends (and of course our own) can sometimes feel overwhelming. If you find these demands unmanageable or unrealistic, consider discussing them and seeking support from those around you.

Connect with Others

Connecting with the community can be a vital way to manage stress. The hashtag #ActuallyAutistic, created in 2011, was designed to provide online space for autistic individuals. Whether online or in person, finding and connecting with other autistic people can significantly aid in coping and provide valuable support. See www.autism.org.uk for more ideas.

www.jeremysachs.com   @JeremySachs_

For A4 and printable versions of this worksheet, visit www.jeremysachs.com

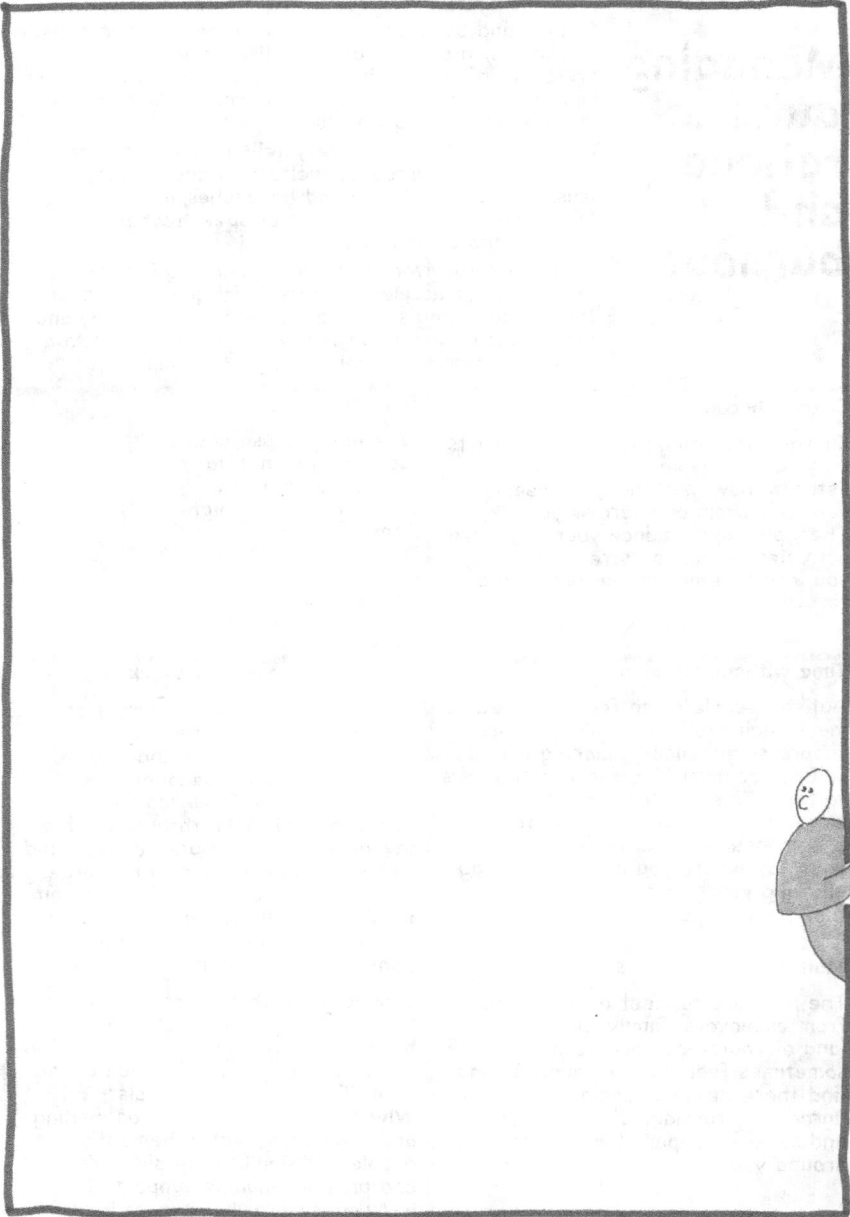

For A4 and printable versions of this worksheet, visit www.jeremysachs.com

Resources

Beyond Betrayal: Taking Charge of Your Life After Boyhood Sexual Abuse by Richard Gartner

ISBN: 9781630260361
This book focuses solely on the topic of betrayal and childhood sexual abuse.

John Bowlby and Attachment Theory: Makers of Modern Psychotherapy by Jeremy Holmes

ISBN 0415629039
This book provides a summary of attachment theory.

Good Will Hunting (1997)

This film focuses on male relationships. The protagonist, Will, struggles with attachment.

Signposting

The ManKind Initiative

https://mankind.org.uk
The ManKind Initiative is a charity that helps men escape domestic violence.

Notes

1 Peter A. Hancock, Deborah R Billings, Kristin E Schaefer, Jessie Y C Chen, Ewart J de Visser, Raja Parasuraman, 'A meta-analysis of factors impacting trust in human-robot interaction', *Human Factors* 53, no. 5 (October 2011): 517–527, doi: 10.1177/0018720811417254.
2 Erik H. Erikson, *Childhood and Society*, 2nd ed. (New York: W.W. Norton & Company, 1993), 247.
3 Erik H. Erikson, *Insight and Responsibility* (New York: W.W. Norton & Company, 1964), 115.
4 'Nature of child sexual abuse: Risk factors & dynamics', Bravehearts, 2024. https://bravehearts.org.au/research-lobbying/stats-facts/nature-of-child-sexual-abuse-risk-factors-dynamics, accessed 2 August 2024.
5 Marc Allroggen, Thea Rau, Jeannine Ohlert, and Jörg M. Fegert, 'Lifetime prevalence and incidence of sexual victimization of adolescents in institutional care', *Child Abuse and Neglect*, no. 66 (April 2017): 23–30, doi: 10.1016/j.chiabu.2017.02.015.
6 Victims' Commissioner, *Annual Report of the Victims' Commissioner, 2021 to 2022* (London: Victims' Commissioner, 2022), 17.
7 Bedbible Research Center, 'Pornhub statistics: Analysis of +9,000 hours of porn', Bedbible, updated 1 May 2024. https://bedbible.com/pornhub-statistics, accessed 2 August 2024.

8   Ateret Gewirtz-Meydan, Denise Volman-Pampanel, Eugenia Opuda, and Noam Tarshish, 'Dating apps: A new emerging platform for sexual harassment? A scoping review', *Trauma, Violence and Abuse* 25, no. 1 (January 2024): 752–763, doi: 10.1177/15248380231162969.

9   Samantha G. Echevarria, Roselyn Peterson, and Jacqueline Woerner, 'College students' experiences of dating app facilitated sexual violence and associations with mental health symptoms and well-being', *Journal of Sex Research* 60, no. 8 (October 2023): 1193–1205, doi: 10.1080/00224499.2022.2130858.

10 Alexis Jay, Malcolm Evans, Ivor Frank, and Drusilla Sharpling, *Child Protection in Religious Organisations and Settings 2021* (The Independent Inquiry into Child Sexual Abuse, September 2021).

11 Kate Dawson, Siobhán Healy-Cullen, Pádraig MacNeela, and Richard de Visser, *An Exploratory Study on Teacher Perpetrated Sexual Misconduct in Irish and UK Secondary Schools*, v. 1 (University of Greenwich, July 2023), 13. https://docs.gre.ac.uk/__data/assets/pdf_file/0027/331398/dawson-29th-august-2023.pdf, accessed 2 August 2024.

12 *The Residential Schools Investigation Report* (The Independent Inquiry into Child Sexual Abuse, 2024). www.iicsa.org.uk/reports-recommendations/publications/investigation/residential-schools/part-k-conclusions-and-recommendations/k1-conclusions.html, accessed 2 August 2024.

13 Revolt Sexual Assault and the Student Room, 'National consultation into the sexual assault and harassment experienced or witnessed by students and graduates from universities across the UK', Revolt Sexual Assault, March 2018. https://revoltsexualassault.com/wp-content/uploads/2018/03/Report-Sexual-Violence-at-University-Revolt-Sexual-Assault-The-Student-Room-March-2018.pdf, accessed 2 August 2024.

14 Care Quality Commission, *Sexual Safety on Mental Health Wards* (London: Care Quality Commission, 2018). www.cqc.org.uk/publications/major-report/sexual-safety-mental-health-wards, accessed 2 August 2024.

15 R.C. Kessler, A. Sonnega, E. Brommet, M. Hughes, and C.B. Nelson, 'Posttraumatic stress disorder in the National Comorbidity Survey', *Archives of General Psychiatry* 52, no. 12 (December 1995): 1048–1060, doi: 10.1001/archpsyc.1995.03950240066012.

16 Raluca M. Gaher, Carol O'Brien, Paul Smiley, and Austin M. Hahn, Alexithymia, coping styles, and traumatic stress symptoms in a sample of veterans who experienced military sexual trauma. *Stress and Health* 23, no. 1 (February 2016): 55–62, doi: 10.1002/smi.2578.

17 Valerie Jenness, Cheryl L. Maxson, Kristy N. Matsuda, and Jennifer Macy Sumner, 'Violence in California correctional facilities: An empirical examination of sexual assault', *The Bulletin* 2, no. 2 (June 2007): 1–4, https://cpb-us-e2.wpmucdn.com/sites.uci.edu/dist/0/1149/files/2013/06/BulletinVol2Issue2.pdf, accessed 2 August 2024.

Chapter 9

Disclosure

The why, when, and how

Chapter Contents

Disclosure

Disclosure is such a broad topic. Within itself [it] includes themes like 'relationships' or 'sex, sexuality, gender'. The abuse has, in one way or another, affected every significant relationship in my life, from friends to family, university and work, medical staff, as well as my relationship to strangers. Being in control of who I tell was the start of addressing it and learning to live alongside, instead of against, myself. Although it's been challenging at times to tell someone close to me about it, it has always been worthwhile and has served to bolster the strength of those relationships that are positive and healing for me.

Group therapy was really helpful to this end though, towards [the] end of group, I learned that [my abuser] had children. I couldn't stop thinking about it and began to feel an urge or drive to report what I'd experienced to the police. I don't regret my decision [to report], but the honest account is that it's a lot. For scale, I just got suddenly made redundant during a cost-of-living crisis, and that feels like absolutely nothing compared with the following two months I have left to wait for the trial, which is ultimately the end result of eventually reporting.

It follows you everywhere, through everything. Intrusive thoughts about silly things like what you'll wear [in court] on the day; or how you'll feel when you see him for the first time, and in a court room, after so many years; police requests from the defence lawyers, when you're on holiday or at Christmastime; requests for your phone or the content of your social media and medical history. Too much contact or not enough – you're never

---

DOI: 10.4324/9781003423331-9

satisfied. And you're only allowed to know so much for the integrity of the case. It can feel like there's no reprieve. So much for such a low conviction rate. I sometimes hear that bravery is knowing you're probably not going to win, that it might even hurt, but you do that thing anyway because it's the right thing to do. I think this may just be heartwarming gibberish, but maybe there's also a room for heartwarming gibberish.

But even so, even with all the meditation and reframing in the world, there's no getting around the likely outcome of the trial, as well as the pain I know I'll go through when I go there. Still, I remind myself that [my abuser] has to go too. He has to hear me and see me and be seen by others. This is the only real guarantee I can rely on. I can't really prepare for it in any traditional sense, but I can prepare how I'm going to manage it. I have to reframe my understanding of what justice is, as if reflecting on the meaning of justice is a normal pastime. And then writing about it for a book, as if that's normal. Though, given the numbers, it's a bit more normal than we might like to think. It's absurd, trying to accept the absurd.

It's not just one thing. It's like a rope. Many strands altogether, overlapping and interlocking, affecting a life. But talking about it, wherever that might lead, is a great way to start untangling

Arthur, gay, trans man

9.1 Disclosure can be hard!

For those whose lives have *not* been affected by trauma, stigma, or misunderstanding, disclosure might not seem complicated. Something happens to you, you tell someone. If you break your leg, you tell a doctor. Next, you call work to say you can't come in; then you ask a friend to do your food shopping and, depending on how good a friend they are, scratch your toes when you can't reach them. The idea of 'disclosing' a broken leg seems overblown; in most cases of a broken leg, you just tell someone, right?

So why dedicate whole chapter to disclosure? A clue may lie in the word's origins. A quick online search tells us the word *disclosure* comes from an old French word, *desclos*, meaning 'open, exposed, explicit'. To people living with HIV, people convicted of a crime, sex workers, or anyone living with an identity that society stigmatises, sharing that part of themselves can feel deeply exposing. Being explicit about our experience or identity can leave us vulnerable to judgement and even violence. This can not only affect us psychologically, but it can also affect employment opportunities, family life, or access to healthcare. Sexual abuse certainly carries huge stigma, and for men who live with this experience, the risks of disclosure can feel life-altering.

Disclosure isn't simply telling another person about abuse; it is exposing one of our most painful experiences to another person and managing any number of their potential responses. The emotional burden of speaking those words – 'I was abused' – is huge, and that is only part of the stress, because survivors are often left managing the emotional reaction of the person disclosed to, which can be another emotional burden. Men have shared stories with me about disclosing sexual abuse to police officers who rolled their eyes or laughed. They've told me stories about disclosing to their wife, only to be told to stop because she won't find them sexy anymore. Trans men who tell their doctors, only to have their T therapy stopped. Friends who learn about the abuse and become inconsolable, taking up all the emotional space. Through misunderstanding, strong reactions, myths, and prejudice, disclosing abuse can harm survivors.

Disclosing abuse can feel so big and dangerous, some survivors wait years before coming forward. This can mean waiting until the perpetrator dies or the survivor moves away. In these cases, outsiders may ask, 'Why did they wait to tell someone?' or the more shaming version, 'They are telling people now because they want something'. Survivors who wait to disclose may be accused of making up sexual abuse for personal gain, attention, or money. This is especially true when the perpetrator is famous or a community leader, like a religious or public figure or someone with responsibility or influence. Some years ago, in an effort to combat such accusations, I drew the comic below to illustrate some of the reasons survivors wait to come forward after abuse. If you're struggling to answer the doubtful or shaming questions or accusations of someone in your life, it may help to share the comic with them. You can tell them which bits feel like they represent your experience or use it as a conversation starter.

TRIGGERING SUBJECT

If you think issues in this support sheet might upset you, make sure to show yourself good self care. Make sure you are somewhere safe, find a friend to read it with or make yourself a big mug of tea.

WHY SOME SEXUAL ABUSE SURVIVORS WAIT TO COME FORWARD

INTRODUCTION

We often hear about survivors of sexual abuse coming forward years after an assault, or after the perpetrator has died.

It can be difficult to understand why the survivor didn't come forward at the time.

Here are some reasons why people wait to come forward.

DANGER

Perpetrators are rarely dodgy looking men in big coats. They are family members, trusted community leaders, or people in positions of power. Some perpetrators show love and care toward young people or earn the trust of a parent or carer.

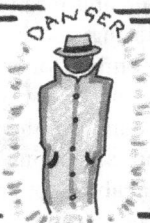

As children we are hardwired to trust adults; it's a survival instinct. It is too unsettling for a child to believe an adult could hurt them or be wrong.

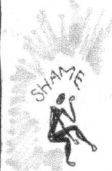

SHAME

Many Perpetrators create a culture of secrecy with a young person. This secrecy, along with trusting an adult not to be 'in the wrong' often leads to feelings of shame developing in the young person.

This can be devastating to their development.

This shame can stay with a young person well into their adulthood, and gives the Perpetrator power over that person. Survivors carry this shame like a heavy dark secret. Society's attitudes to survivors, whatever their gender identity, can be blaming and add more shame; often it can feel safer to keep quiet.

After a Perpetrator dies, often their power dies with them and survivors feel free to disclose their experiences — we have seen this in many of the high profile cases in the news over the last few years.

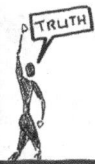

TRUTH

It has been estimated that the average male survivor takes 26 years to tell anyone they have been abused.

www.jeremysachs.com   @JeremySachs_

For A4 and printable versions of this worksheet, visit www.jeremysachs.com

If disclosure is so risky, why disclose at all? It might seem better to keep sexual abuse a secret and never risk telling anyone. Arthur's testimony at the beginning of this chapter puts it beautifully: 'Being in control of who I tell was the start of addressing it and learning to live alongside, instead of against, myself'. Disclosing can be the start of addressing the trauma of sexual abuse and learning how to manage it, instead of being managed by it. Disclosing can help us put words to the abuse and start to put the blame and shame we feel where it belongs: on the perpetrator. Practically, disclosing can help explain to others some of the challenges we experience and communicate the support we need. It can be the first step towards receiving some form of justice or towards connecting with people in our world in an emotionally authentic way.

Connecting to people

We need connections in our lives like we need air. As social creatures, we cannot thrive without connecting to people. It is an evolutionary imperative to build bonds with others. On the other hand, as survivors, we have needed to develop complex defence mechanisms, some of which can isolate us rather than connecting us. These defence mechanisms can include anything from taking a long time to trust people to using drugs, work, alcohol, or sex to avoid meaningful relationships. We may also develop an aggressive or sarcastic persona to keep people at a distance. Despite these mechanisms keeping us isolated, we may find ourselves desperately wanting someone to know what we survived. Still, sexual abuse is difficult – we want people to know, but we don't want to talk about it. Additionally, some people don't want to hear about it, too uncomfortable to sit with or think about abuse. This dynamic can make conversations about abuse feel vulnerable for everyone.

Disclosing to a family member may mean navigating lots of complicated history and emotions. If the abuse happened in childhood, for example, you may need to consider whether the family member you wish to tell knew or still knows the perpetrator. It is rare that children meet people who are completely separate from their family. Perpetrators are often family members or people close to the family, such as friends or community figures. The family member you want to disclose to could experience complicated emotions towards the perpetrator as well as towards you, the survivor. They may be close to the perpetrator and need to go through their own journey of anger or grief over that relationship. They could also feel guilt for failing to protect you or notice that something was wrong. Victim blaming can also occur within families; when the idea of a loved one abusing a child is too emotionally difficult, some may blame or ignore the survivor instead.

Disclosing abuse that occurred in adulthood can be challenging for different reasons. If the abuse happened on a night out or at a chemsex party, survivors may also need to consider how or whether to disclose sexuality or drug use. This may open us up to victim blaming or disbelief from family or friends who do not believe adult men can be victims of sexual abuse or rape and who don't take it seriously.

They may accuse the survivor of having sex outside a marriage or relationship, or they may not acknowledge the power of sexual assault or the lack of consent involved. Some people may demand more information than we are willing to share, which can become highly stressful. Survivors who want to disclose to a partner or spouse may encounter blaming or shaming, which can be emasculating and render the wounds of abuse even more painful.

Starting new sexual relationships can feel enormously vulnerable. Men commonly feel pressure to want sex or to perform well sexually. Members of stereotyped groups, such as gay men, can be expected to have many sexual partners whereas Black men can be expected to be sexually assertive. Some survivors will feel these stereotyped expectations acutely, almost always leading to problems. Male survivors of all backgrounds who want to start having sex with a new partner may find that we are not starting from neutral. Our new partner may already have sexual expectations of us (assertiveness, always being up for sex, dominance, experience etc), and this can make disclosing sexual trauma especially difficult. Some men avoid disclosing but, by doing so, risk having a trauma response, such as freezing or running away, before, during, or after sex. The fear of disclosure and its consequences can be so profound, survivors may find ourselves stuck in a pattern of behaviour where we seek sexual or emotional connection, only to be retraumatised and isolate ourselves. Once isolated, we again seek sexual or emotional connection, and the pattern repeats (for more on sex, see page 130).

The battle between our desire to connect to people and our fear of disclosure is one of the hardest we have to fight, and it's one many of us have to repeat often throughout our lives. This is because disclosure doesn't happen only once. New relationships, therapists and friends bring new scenarios where we may choose to disclose. Ultimately as humans, we have a primal instinct to grow towards others, regardless of whether or not we experience abuse. Because all humans do this, I believe it is possible for all of us to find people to whom we'll be able to disclose in a way that feels connective and allows us space to tell our stories and heal.

9.2   The authorities: Friend or foe?

A vast majority of the dialogue around seeking justice after sexual abuse focuses on disclosure and reporting criminal cases to the police, in other words, it focuses on punishing abusers. But survivors can seek to disclose in other forms of justice. In the following sections, we'll look at criminal law, civil law, anonymous reporting, and transformative justice (TJ) (also covered in Chapter 11, page 217). It is especially useful to know a bit about different types of reporting for survivors who feel uncomfortable with the criminal justice system due to immigration status, previous experiences, or fear of persecution. Knowing your options is important.

In 2022, I interviewed Claire Waxman, the London victims' commissioner, for an episode of my podcast, *The Trauma Talks*. It's Claire's job to overhaul the criminal justice system, campaign on behalf of crime victims, and ensure they have agency over what happens, regardless of whether or not they report the abuse as a crime. We talked about disclosing abuse to the authorities and police attitudes towards male survivors. She told me,

> Police practice still needs to drastically improve in this area, and we need to see better training. We need to expand police officers' knowledge, and we really need to tackle this culture that is including too many assumptions and prejudice and biases that are preventing and causing real barriers for justice and support for male victims.
>
> I want to encourage victims and survivors to come forward, but I don't want them to come forward into a system that will retraumatise them and will compound their trauma and make it far harder for them to cope and recover and survive in their day-to-day.... We do know, unfortunately, a survivor may get the wrong response from a police officer that may well make their trauma much worse.[1]

For decades, significant parts of the British population, particularly LGBTQIA+ and ethnic minority communities, have known that the police as an organisation could retraumatise survivors. In 1981, for example, the Brixton riots resulted from racist discrimination towards the Black community, perpetrated mainly by white police officers. In 1993, 18-year-old Stephen Lawrence was killed in a racially motivated attack at a bus stop. Eighteen years later, the report into the police investigation showed it had been 'marred by a combination of professional incompetence, institutional racism and a failure of leadership'.[2] Often, police failure has been explained away as the result of 'a few bad apples' – that only a small number of individual officers were responsible for prejudice and abuse, and the police force as a whole was open and inclusive. Police remained in denial of institutional abusive practices until *The Baroness Casey Review* was published in 2023, following the kidnap, rape, and murder of Sarah Everard by a serving Metropolitan Police (Met) officer.

The report found the Met to be institutionally racist, misogynist, and homophobic, with widespread bullying. It found 'deep-seated homophobia within the Met' – many LGBTQIA+ Met employees reported personally experiencing homophobia, and 30 per cent of LGBTQIA+ employees reported being bullied. Female officers and staff 'routinely face sexism and misogyny.'[3] The Met is the UK's largest police force. It's easy to see why male survivors of sexual abuse may hesitate to disclose to police anywhere in the United Kingdom.

Some survivors of sexual abuse may face compounding vulnerabilities due to their intersecting identities, such as being Black, gay, transgender, or working class. These intersections can increase survivors' susceptibility to police discrimination. Seeking support from the police can result in further trauma if survivors encounter oppression or discrimination. Even men who do not belong to a minority community or have a marginalised identity may face significant challenges when reporting to the authorities, including stigma, belittling, incompetence, or a generally upsetting experience.

Until the early 2020s, many men experienced these challenges without professional or emotional support. For much of history, survivors in the UK were advised against seeking therapy or specialist services while their cases were in court because notes from therapists could be admitted as evidence, violating confidentiality. Crown Prosecution Service guidelines warned that therapy might lead to allegations of coaching by the defence, which could be used against survivors in court. This changed in May 2023, with amendments to the Victims and Prisoners Bill that protect the privacy of survivors' therapy sessions. Prior to this, survivors had to pursue justice with minimal or no therapeutic support, making it even more challenging to manage their trauma and emotional recovery.

Despite all of these challenges, men do report to the police. Some have a negative experience, and some have a positive one. This disparity is upsetting. It can feel so unfair that I struggled with including this section in the book. How could I, in good conscience, signpost survivors to a potentially retraumatising institution? In the end, I included the information because of all the men I have supported who have had positive experiences with police, but I want to make it clear that I respect and believe survivors whose experience with police led to further traumatisation. The end of this chapter includes signposting to a variety of alternative forms of reporting to give survivors as much agency as possible.

Ultimately, it is your choice whether or not to report. Sexual abuse and rape remove our agency and ability to consent. For this reason, it is especially important that you have total agency over if, when, and to whom you report. For now, here is some practical information that should give you an idea of what to expect when reporting to the police. Keep in mind, however, that this process may change in the future or be different depending on the country you're in.

Deciding whether to report to police

There are no rights or wrongs about reporting; it is important to do what is right for you. Some survivors feel it is very important to report sexual abuse or assault, historical or recent, to the police. Others do not wish to consider it. Still others feel it is a more complex decision.

Here are some reasons survivors give for reporting:

- It was a crime, and the perpetrator should be brought to justice.
- I want the perpetrator to be held accountable.
- I want to ensure that it doesn't happen again to someone else.
- I don't want it to be a secret anymore.
- I want to speak my truth.
- I want to punish the perpetrator, and this is a legal way of doing that.
- I want the perpetrator to know I remember what they did.
- I want to stand up for something I believe is right.
- The police have contacted me out of the blue because someone else has reported.

Here are some reasons survivors give for not reporting:

- Given the circumstances of the abuse, it is unlikely the perpetrator will be convicted.
- It would cause damage to people I love.
- I have ambivalent or loving feelings towards the perpetrator and don't want to cause them harm.
- I don't want to put myself through it.
- I do not know who the perpetrator is.
- I cannot trust the police because:
  - I am an asylum-seeker and fearful how reporting may affect my status.
  - I fear the police may further endanger my safety because of my identity or experience.
  - I'm a sex worker, and the police do not acknowledge my experience as a rape.
  - I was doing something illegal when I was assaulted.
- It happened in another country, and it's unlikely to come to anything.
- The perpetrator is dead, and it doesn't feel like there is any point.

These are not exhaustive lists. It can be helpful to consider why you may or may not choose to report the abuse you experienced. Take some time to make a list of both reasons *to* and *not to* report. Decide what feels most important for you.

Being outed

Sometimes, when a survivor makes an allegation of sexual abuse and names other potential survivors, the police may contact those other survivors to give evidence, even though they did not report (and, in some cases, have never even disclosed the abuse). Feeling pressure to give evidence to strengthen another survivor's case can feel particularly difficult when we haven't chosen to go to the police ourselves. It can be even harder if the other survivor is known to us.

Some countries have what's called mandatory reporting laws for sexual abuse, and teachers, therapists, or social workers are by law obligated to make a report when we mention abuse to them. This looks different from country to country, but it can be distressing for survivors, particularly those in therapy. It takes survivors a huge amount of bravery to tell any part of our story. When therapists are compelled to break confidentiality or advise us to not disclose information lest they need to escalate, it can retraumatise survivors. A study conducted at University College Cork in Ireland was published in 2022. As Seán Pellegrini, lead researcher of the 2022 study 'Experiences of psychologists in applying mandatory reporting in Ireland (Children First)', told journalists,

While participants believed that Mandatory Reporting was introduced with well-meaning and good intentions, they noted how they felt that it has paradoxically put people at increased risk.

Psychologists in the current research described how clients who did not wish to participate in the Mandatory Reporting process could not discuss certain traumas as this would have automatically triggered a referral.

One psychologist in the study said, 'I know that there is all this stuff that they're not telling me because they know I would have to report it, and it tends to be key information.'[4]

It is important to know that, even when police contact you, it is still your choice whether or not to give evidence.

Reporting to police

You can report an abuse or rape to the police in person, online, or via telephone. Rape Crisis, a UK charity that supports survivors, advise that, if the abuse or rape is recent, police should check that you are safe and whether you need any medical support. They may also want to collect forensic evidence, which may include anything from bodily fluids to clothing fabrics from the perpetrator. It may help the police collect this evidence if you do not

- Eat or drink
- Smoke
- Wash or comb your hair
- Change clothing
- Move or clean anything where the rape or assault happened

Needless to say, it can be hard not to do these things (for a comprehensive list, see https://rapecrisis.org.uk). If you have done some or all of them, that's okay too; you can still make a report (see signposting for rape crisis links at the end of the chapter, page 190).

Police may also ask if you want to do a forensic medical exam. In the UK, this normally takes place at a sexual assault referral centre (SARC). Even if you don't want to report right now, you can still go to a SARC and allow them to collect evidence. They will store it for you until you are ready to report. Some SARCs also offer sexual health and counselling services. They have advice and are generally comfortable places designed for people of all genders and ages. If the assault or rape happened a while ago or in childhood, you won't have to go to a SARC or give forensic evidence. Even though you cannot provide evidence of historical abuse, the police should still count your testimony as evidence and investigate, no matter how long ago the assault was.

The first report is an initial account of what happened. Police won't ask for in-depth details straight away. At this point, they just want enough to get the ball rolling. If possible, depending on where you are, they may also assign a specialist police officer with training in sexual offences and working with survivors.

Giving a statement

After you report, the police will want to take an official statement, usually recorded by video (not just audio, like in films and TV). If your case goes to court, this recorded video may be used as testimony. You can ask for a male or female police officer and have a friend or loved one support you, if you like. After you give your statement, the police must make (often extensive) enquiries to determine whether there is sufficient evidence to take the perpetrator to court. They may contact the perpetrator and interview people you know. This period can be lengthy, sometimes taking one or two years.

Going to criminal court

Often with abuse crimes, there are few or no witnesses. Frustratingly, this can mean there is insufficient evidence to bring the case to court. This can be extremely upsetting to survivors who have decided to disclose. It is really important to remember that even if a case does not make it to court, it does not mean that people don't believe you or that the abuse did not happen or was not serious. It just means that it is unlikely a conviction would be secured because there is a lack of hard evidence.

If the case does go to court, there can still be lots of waiting. This can give survivors time to consider some important support strategies. Consider the following questions:

- Who am I going to tell about the court case?
- Do I want someone to come with me? If so, do I want them to come into the court room? What might they learn about my experience? Would I prefer for them to stay in the waiting area until afterwards?
- How can I support myself emotionally if I am cross-examined by the perpetrator's defence lawyer?
- What do I need to do before and after the court to look after myself?
- What if I want to pull out of the whole thing? How might that feel, and how will I look after myself?
  (NOTE: Keep in mind, you can always pull out of the case; however, the case may still go ahead if the police feel there is enough evidence to convict).
- How will I feel if there is a conviction? How will I feel if there is not a conviction?
  (NOTE: It's worth considering how you will feel and cope whether or not the perpetrator is found guilty. Remember, if they are found not guilty, it doesn't mean that the sexual assault or abuse didn't happen. It just means there was not enough hard evidence to convict. If the perpetrator is found guilty, it may be a relief, or you may have more complicated or ambivalent feelings. Whatever you feel is OK).

Other ways of seeking justice

Civil law

The criminal court procedure I just described is the type we most often think of when we think about the law. Criminal courts are used to prove guilt and punish people who commit crimes. Civil law is an alternative to this procedure. Civil courts do not seek criminal conviction, and cases don't always end up going to court. Civil law seeks compensation for wrongdoing from the defendant or perpetrator, rather than punishment. Civil law varies across the four UK nations, but depending on where you live and the circumstances of the abuse, sexual abuse may come under the category of 'trespass to the person', for which survivors can seek compensation in civil court. The burden of evidence also differs between the two. Criminal court requires evidence 'beyond all reasonable doubt', but civil courts only require that the claimant prove their case based on the balance of probabilities. This means that the available evidence suggests the claim is more likely than not to be true.

Anonymous reporting

Anonymous reporting is informing the police about the abuse without giving them your personal information or making an official report. This type of reporting can put the perpetrator on the police's radar, but it may not lead to an arrest. In addition, because the police do not have your personal information, they will not contact you to inform you what action they take based on your report.

While some survivors feel like reporting anonymously leads to little or no police action, it helps others feel like the abuse has less power over them. It may help survivors feel safer if they worry the perpetrator has access to vulnerable people. If the perpetrator is already known to the police, anonymous reports can help them build their profile and better look out for sexual abuse towards others.

Transformative justice (TJ)

TJ is a political framework designed to create positive change within our society and communities. It aims to end cycles of violence and abuse in our communities. It nurtures accountability, healing, and safety for all, in particular, helping survivors to heal from the damage of harm. TJ also works to end the root causes of sexual abuse and violence, such as generational trauma, poverty, misogyny, ableism, and oppression of people from minority backgrounds. Practically, this will look different depending on your circumstances and engagement with TJ. In the therapy world, it is a relatively new concept, about which I talk more in Chapter 11.

9.3   Taking back power

All disclosures differ from one another. What works for one situation might not for another. Disclosing to police will feel different compared to disclosing to a parent. Disclosing to a parent will feel different compared to disclosing to a new sexual partner.

Sometimes, as survivors feel more empowered and in control of our life and story, we can 'over-disclose' and regret sharing our experience, or so much of it. This can result in shameful feelings and anxiety that the information we give people about our experience can come back and harm us in the future.

Reflective activity

Because of the discrepancies between different types of disclosure, it's impossible to provide a step-by-step guide that suits every situation. Instead, I have created a list of ideas to consider and questions to ask yourself. Hopefully, these will help you decide how and whether to disclose in any situation you come across.

Who

Who do you want to tell? Are they likely to tell someone else (a partner, for example)? Are you okay with this? Can they be trusted with your story? Will you be glad you told them one month from now?

Work out who you *don't* want to know about this information. This may be particularly important if disclosing to a member of a family or social group. People naturally want to share big information. Make your boundaries around your story clear.

What

You do not have to disclose everything. This sounds obvious, but once we start talking, it is sometimes difficult to censor ourselves. Sometimes, just telling a loved one the abuse happened is enough. Decide which details you want to share and which may be safer to keep private for now.

How

Get practical. Plan the disclosure out in detail. Will you do it in your own home, on a walk, in a cafe? Think about the environment you will need both during the disclosure and afterwards. The time of day may be important, as well. Allow time afterwards to process the experience and do something completely different to decompress.

Even if your disclosure ends up completely different from how you planned it, having a plan can manage your anxiety.

When

When is it best to tell someone? A busy public holiday or celebration with lots of friends and family around may be a terrible idea for some, but it may feel really supportive for others. Everyone will be different and require different environments.

Why

Consider why you are choosing to tell your story now. What do *you* want to gain? What happens if you don't get what you want from the disclosure? You cannot control other people's reactions, nor are you responsible for them. You may feel disappointed if the moment doesn't feel liberating or the person you confide in does not respond in the way you want. Hope for a positive experience, but by all means, consider what you will need if it goes poorly.

Safety

If you are still connected to the abuser, such as within a group or environment, telling someone in that group or environment may be a risk. It is critical to ensure your physical safety is not compromised by disclosing. If you feel like you are at risk, it is essential you find a professional to speak to. This could be the police, but for those who do not want to speak to the police, one safe potential first step to getting long-term support is to contact an independent sexual violence adviser or anonymous helpline. Protecting your mental health is important, too. Have a safety plan for after the disclosure, including experiences or objects that make you feel safe.

As we've discussed, disclosure is not something we do once and never again. As our life goes on, we meet new people and find ourselves in new situations, such as new jobs or relationships, in which we need to decide whether to disclose and what we may gain or risk. Our feelings about the abuse and ourselves may also change. While disclosing may feel terrifying at first, as we connect with different parts of ourselves and grow emotionally, we may find disclosing less scary or not as big a deal. It can go the other way, too; what might be easy today could become difficult tomorrow. Complicating disclosure even more is the fact that the counselling, psychotherapy, and psychology industries for years have upheld the myth that survivors must talk about sexual trauma in order to heal from it. We know now people can be harmed when clinical professionals or social workers force survivors to disclose. No one has the right to make you share something you do not want to.

I believe in the healing power of disclosure. Being heard and believed is important, but not when you feel uncomfortable disclosing. I also believe you can have healing experiences without disclosing. Many men have sat in my support groups without ever disclosing information about their abuse. At that time in their lives, listening to others and connecting to people who shared their experience was enough. The most important thing is that you choose to tell – or not tell – your story when – and if – you want to. Deciding who you tell and when can be your first step in asking for support, regaining agency over your story and taking back power from those who tried to remove it from you.

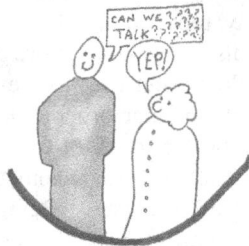

Telling People About Your Abuse

If you're unsure whether to disclose your abuse or how to do so, consider asking yourself these questions to help you think about disclosure. If you have a trusted friend or therapist, you might also discuss this sheet with them.

WHO?	WHAT?	HOW?
Determine who you want to disclose to and who you don't. How can you ensure these boundaries are respected and maintained?	Determine which details you're willing to share and which you want to keep private. Don't feel pressured to share more than you're comfortable with.	Consider how you want to disclose: at home, in public, with a friend, or alone? If face-to-face isn't possible, could you use a letter or email?

WHY?	WHEN?	SAFETY?
Why are you choosing to share your story now? Consider what you might gain compared to the potential risks or disappointments.	When is the best and safest time to tell someone? If there isn't a perfect time, can you create a 'good enough' time?	What if it goes wrong? How will you keep yourself emotionally and/or physically safe, whether from your own reaction or others' responses?

Disclosure is often one of the hardest things anyone can do, especially for men. Take your time and remember, you are in control of your story and what you choose to share or keep private. Plan what you'll do before and after disclosing to ensure you stay safe, comfortable, and well cared for throughout the process.

www.jeremysachs.com   @JeremySachs_

For A4 and printable versions of this worksheet, visit www.jeremysachs.com

www.jeremysachs.com   @JeremySachs_

For A4 and printable versions of this worksheet, visit www.jeremysachs.com

Resources

The Boy with the Perpetual Nervousness: A Memoir of an Adolescence *by Graham Caveney*

ISBN: 9781509830671
This memoir reflects on the author's experiences of growing up working class in Northern England in the 1960s and of sexual abuse perpetrated by a Catholic priest.

Signposting

Crime Stoppers

https://crimestoppers-uk.org
Crime Stoppers is a UK charity that can support survivors reporting anonymously.

Rape Crisis England & Wales and Rape Crisis Scotland

https://rapecrisis.org.uk, www.rapecrisisscotland.org.uk
Rape Crisis is a charity that gives advice on everything from what to do after an assault to finding support.

Notes

1 'Male survivors of abuse in adulthood', *The Trauma Talks*, series 2, episode 1 (Apple Podcasts, 9 May 2023), https://podcasts.apple.com/gb/podcast/2-1-the-trauma-talks-male-survivors-of-sexual-abuse/id1517405491?i=1000612318642, accessed 2 August 2024.
2 William Macpherson, *The Stephen Lawrence Inquiry*, Report of an inquiry by Sir William Macpherson of Cluny, advised by Tom Cook, the right reverend Dr John Sentamu, Dr Richard Stone: presented to Parliament by the Secretary of State for the Home Department by Command of Her Majesty, February 1999. https://assets.publish ing.service.gov.uk/government/uploads/system/uploads/attachment_data/file/277111/4262.pdf, accessed 2 August 2024.
3 Baroness Casey of Blackstock DBE CB, *Baroness Casey Review: Final Report: An Independent Review into the Standards of Behaviour and Internal Culture of the Metropolitan Police Service* (London: Metropolitan Police, March 2023). www.met.police.uk/SysSiteAssets/media/downloads/met/about-us/baroness-casey-review/update-march-2023/baroness-casey-review-march-2023a.pdf, accessed 2 August 2024..
4 Seán Pellegrini, 'Experiences of psychologists in applying mandatory reporting in Ireland (Children First)', *Journal of Public Child Welfare* 17, no. 5 (October 2022): 1086–1109, https://doi.org/10.1080/15548732.2022.2137272.

Chapter 10

Coping

The unsustainable and the sustainable

Chapter Contents

Trauma and the body: A reflection

I am a morbidly obese man. I have had issues with binge eating and body image since I was a teen. I have suffered the health consequences of that as well as the logistical. I have suffered the shame that goes with it, too, every time I have to get in [an] aeroplane seat or walk through a crowded pub. Safe to say, I hate my body. Its folds, its heft, and the fact that to clothe it, I always have to buy online.

I wasn't always this way. I was a relatively normal little boy. Then puberty hit, and I suddenly found myself being abused by a neighbour of my parents. I did not recognise it as abuse at first. I saw it as being 'close', but abuse it was. You would never have known from my demeanour. However, from the age of 13, I began to binge-eat and began to quietly descend into what became a loathing of my body. I did not recognise this as trauma, but I effectively shut myself down. My teen years and then into my twenties saw this hatred of the very skin I inhabited. I was not a natural athlete. I am very short, not especially handsome, and had issues with my genitals from childhood that meant that my response to the abuse was to consider my penis and testicles as not a part of my body. They had let me down. They had reacted with pleasure to something that was anything but. So my body got bigger until, eventually, a plateau was reached, and with the love of a good woman, I began to see myself differently – not as a sexual being, never that – but as someone who had some worth. Then I was raped at the age of 34. My response to this trauma was to disappear inside a fridge and never come out. I went from plump to obese within a few years, not helped by my inability to

DOI: 10.4324/9781003423331-10

tell anyone about what had happened. My eating was the one element of my life I felt able to control. So I did, and I ate when I liked, where I liked, and how much I liked.

It wasn't just the binge eating that exploded as a response to the traumatic events. I lived in a constant state of fear. I did not recognise that for many years. But day to day, I would be taken back to the events, triggered by the smell of grass or the sound of a car on gravel. By plastic bags. By fallen leaves. My body reacted by going cold, but sweating. By finding myself somewhere else and ... freezing at the most inappropriate times.

This cycle of bingeing, triggers, and flashbacks continued for 15-plus years and can still rear its head even now. When I undertook counselling with SurvivorsUK, I would leave the group session on a Saturday morning and head to the McDonalds next door. It gave me control over myself, but of course I wasn't really in control. The self-hatred that came following such a binge was testament to that.

It would be lovely to give this story a happy ending. To say everything is now fine and dandy. That I have a 32 waist and have no flashbacks, that I never binge-eat or use food as an escape. No such luck. I lost my wife to cancer recently, and the trauma of those events showed how little control I have over myself, from eating to the lack of care of myself.

However, not all is doom and gloom. [There are] things I have done right. Seeking help. Counselling. Being open about my experiences. Finding ways to ground myself when experiencing flashbacks. Making sure my feet are firmly on the ground, learning how to meditate and breathe coherently, and realising self-hatred affects no one else but me, so channelling blame where it should go. It's a journey without end. But then again, that is life.

Chris, white, bisexual man, 58

10.1   The nature of coping

As we all know, the aftermath of abuse is challenging. It can be frightening, shameful, infuriating, saddening, and confusing. These strong feelings require survivors to develop coping strategies to manage them, in addition to the struggles of everyday life. There are lots of strategies out there; everyone from social media influencers to healthcare providers offers them. But what happens when the pain we are trying to manage is more powerful than the recommended coping strategy?

I have worked with teenagers frustrated at professionals who suggested a 'hot bath' as a way of coping with sexual abuse. I've talked with men who saw on social media that yoga can help us heal from trauma but never went to a class because the yoga studios near them feel too middle-class, inaccessible to diverse bodies, feminine, expensive, or white. Both of these examples present difficult challenges. A hot bath may not even begin to address the young person's problem (and, in fact, may have made them feel worse), and while yoga *might* help with trauma, if we can't access classes for reasons of identity or money, we are prevented from ever finding out. This can leave survivors with few options when it comes to coping strategies. Instead of taking a hot bath, some survivors may choose to self-harm by cutting themselves because it feels like a stronger, more immediate response to feeling bad. Instead of yoga, some survivors may choose to overeat junk foods, which are more easily accessible to them.

Though it might sound counterintuitive, in the therapy room, I would never say that self-harm or overeating are bad. This is not because I want people to self-harm, but because in my experience, coping strategies are signs that we want to change traumatic and difficult feelings, and a desire to change is often a first step to healing. However, I commonly hear about therapists saying things like, 'While you're actively hurting yourself, I can't work with you'. Though there are many legitimate reasons for a therapist to say this, all too often, survivors feel blamed and shamed hearing this, as if they are too damaged to help.

Psychologist Carl Rogers is largely credited as being one of the founders of humanistic psychotherapy. He is often the first person students learn about when training to become a humanistic or integrative therapist. Rogers believed that all living things have a drive towards growth. According to Rogers, we are all striving forward, trying to reach our full potential. In his 1980 book *A Way of Being*, Rogers, who grew up on a farm, describes watching 'sad, spindly' potato sprouts struggle to grow in his basement:

> The sprouts were, in their bizarre, futile growth, a sort of desperate expression of the directional tendency I have been describing. They would never become plants, never mature, never fulfil their real potential. But under the most adverse circumstances, they were striving to become. Life would not give up, even if it could not flourish. In dealing with clients whose lives have been terribly warped, in working with men and women on the back wards of state hospitals, I often think of those potato sprouts. So unfavourable have been the conditions in which these people have developed that their lives often seem abnormal, twisted, scarcely human. Yet, the directional tendency in them can be trusted. The clue to understanding their behaviour is that they are striving, in the only ways that they perceive as available to them, to move towards growth, towards becoming. To healthy persons, the results may seem bizarre and futile, but they are life's desperate attempt to become itself.[1]

What Rogers is saying is that living things will attempt to better themselves, regardless of the resources available to them. Often, survivors of sexual abuse have not been given many resources in life. Where Rogers' potatoes didn't have good soil, water, or sunlight, survivors often lack safety and the belief of others. We may face intersectional challenges or struggle to find specialised help. This means we have to find alternative ways of coping, and not all of those ways will be considered healthy, socially acceptable, or sustainable.

10.2   The unsustainable

Men trying to manage the pain of sexual abuse can find ourselves backed into a corner. Society wants victims to behave in ways contradictory to how it wants men to behave. 'Real men don't cry' is a common expression and a powerful way to communicate that men are not allowed to be victims. Conventional masculinity does not allow 'weakness' (see Chapter 4, on masculinity, for more, page 62). With nowhere safe and socially acceptable to turn, many male survivors develop unsustainable coping strategies, many of which society uses to further vilifies them. Punching walls, using drugs or alcohol, and emotionally shutting down are often seen as aggressive or emotionally immature rather than desperate attempts to manage emotional pain without resources. The outcome of this can be disastrous. For example, a 2006 study of 100 randomly chosen people in US prisons published in the journal *Child Abuse and Neglect* reported that 59 per cent of respondents had experienced some form of sexual abuse before or at the age of 13. The average age of abuse in the study was nine-and-a-half.[2] A 2019 NHS study of 468 males in Welsh prisons found that 8 in 10 reported experiencing at least one ACE, and nearly half had experienced four or more ACEs, including sexual abuse. Drug offences were the second most common type of crime committed by the men in the study, at 53.4 per cent, eclipsed only by theft, at 54.9 per cent.[3] It's important not to assume that sexual abuse predetermines drug use or prison, but when we try and understand the lives of many of the most vulnerable men in society, sexual abuse is often one piece of the puzzle.

The trauma lens

The harm of sexual abuse can obscure how we process thoughts and experiences. We see everything, including ourselves, through a trauma lens, which can affect our core beliefs about ourselves. It's common for men to believe things like

• I am a bad and untrustworthy person who will always let people down.
• Even people who know me don't know the 'real' me, and if they did, they would be disgusted.
• I am damaged goods, and nothing and no one can help.
• If I am going to get better, I must do it on my own.
• I deserve my unsustainable coping strategy, be it self-harm, nicotine, cheating, substance misuse etc.

This trauma lens affects not only our beliefs about ourselves but also our beliefs about the interactions in our lives. It even taints seemingly mundane interactions. Experiencing this every day can reinforce our negative core beliefs. Here are some elements of our everyday lives that the trauma lens can taint:

- **How we interpret other people's actions or words.** We may feel that people are always out to get us or that we're not liked or respected. Even friends we have known for a long time may seem threatening. We may spend hours going over social interactions, from conversations to text messages, trying to interpret what people mean and how they feel about us.
- **How we find meaning in life events that happen to us.** We may feel like bad things, big or small, always happen to us. We may feel personally attacked at every red traffic light or cancelled train. Every negative event can feel personally designed to challenge or hurt us.
- **How we make sense of past relationships or look for new ones.** We may feel like we are always attracted to people who are bad for us. It may feel like the wrong, or even abusive, people somehow spot us a mile off. It can sometimes feel like we deserve these bad relationships while at other times, we may tell ourselves if we can just make it work, or fix this one person, then we'll be happy.
- **How we view our worth in different situations, like relationships or work.** Sexual trauma can leave us believing we are not worthy of respect in all parts of our lives. If someone used us when we were vulnerable, we may believe we do not deserve respect and good things in life. We may learn to expect the worst from careers and the people around us. We may become content with the bare minimum.
- **How we prioritise our wellbeing.** If we feel like the world does not respect us or take us seriously, it can be easy to stop prioritising our own wellbeing. This may mean partaking in behaviour that hurts our loved ones or neglecting our physical health or personal hygiene. If we do not feel that we have worth in the world, why would we be bothered to take care of ourselves?

Thanks to the trauma lens, survivors often struggle to believe that we deserve help or positive relationships. We can develop relationships with compulsive behaviours or addictions rather than loved ones because they don't make the same demands of us that human relationships do. We may feel that we deserve a relationship with drugs or alcohol, rather than relationships with people who want to love and care for us.

Reflective activity

Many negative beliefs we have about ourselves or our world can be summed up by Cognitive Distortions. Take a look at this worksheet and see if any of these apply to how you think about yourself:

Catastrophising:
Believing that the worst possible outcome will happen, and nothing else is possible.

Personalisation:
Blaming yourself unnecessarily for external negative events, even when you may only be partly or not responsible at all.

'Should' Statements:
Focusing on how you believe things 'should' or 'must' be, rather than how it is.

'I should be able to feel better by myself'.

Blaming:
This is like the opposite of personalisation. Blaming takes no responsibility for a negative situation, and puts all blame on someone or something else.

Magnification:
Exaggerating a mistake, or a quality in yourself so it is disproportionately negative.

'I am the worst person in the World'.

Jumping To Conclusions:
Making a statement or conclusion without knowing if there is evidence to support it. These statements are often based on a feeling we have, rather than facts or evidence.

Minimisation:
Seeing your strengths, qualities and accomplishments as small and unimportant.

'The new job is no big deal'.

Mind Reading:
This can be similar to 'jumping to conclusions' where we assume we know what someone else is thinking.

Emotional Reasoning:
Believing that because we feel something, it must be true.

'I feel like a bad father; therefore I must be a bad father'.

Fortune Telling:
Much like 'jumping to conclusions' where we make predictions about what is going to happen in the future, most commonly, negative predictions.

Mental Filter:
When we focus on only one aspect of a situation, often negative, and ignore the rest, often positive.

Overgeneralisation:
Using a single negative event, and applying it to all future situations.

I ALWAYS MESS UP

YOU NEVER LISTEN TO ME

Black & White Thinking:
Seeing things as all good or all bad – one extreme or the other, there are no in-between.

Labelling:
Giving a general label to ourselves or others based on a specific situation.

Disqualifying the Positive:
A mental filter where we dismiss the positive things about ourselves or our life because we believe it doesn't count.

These are **Cognitive Distortions.** They involve negative thinking patterns, or biases, that aren't based on fact or reality. Over time we can become stuck, believing they are true about any number of situations or interactions.

www.jeremysachs.com @JeremySachs_

For A4 and printable versions of this worksheet, visit www.jeremysachs.com

Catching Your Cognitive Distortions

Cognitive distortions are powerful ways of thinking that can hold us back, impact our mood, and affect our relationships. They are powerful because we often learn them early in life, and it can be difficult to unlearn patterns that have been with us for most of our lives. The next time you catch yourself using one of the cognitive distortions mentioned on the previous page, here are six things you can try to take away their power.

(1) Look for patterns

Look for patterns in the way you think and feel. Do you often tell yourself you're 'useless' or that 'other people don't respect you'? Try to identify the repetitive thoughts or beliefs you have about yourself or the world around you.

(2) Challenge automatic thoughts

Challenge automatic thoughts when they arise. The next time you catch yourself thinking or saying an automatic thought, look for evidence that supports it. Ask yourself if the situation is more nuanced than it seems.

(3) Imagine an alternative

Imagine an alternative where your automatic thoughts or patterns aren't the only possible outcome. Could there be a different, less challenging or difficult result? Consider other possibilities that might be more balanced or constructive.

(4) Practise distancing

Practise distancing yourself from harmful labels or self-beliefs. The next time you're hard on yourself, try speaking to yourself as you would to a friend in distress, offering compassion, understanding, and patience instead.

(5) When stuck, move

When stuck, move your body. move your body, If you find yourself caught in a cycle of cognitive distortion, try doing something physical to shift your focus. Walk, stretch, roll your shoulders— even changing the room you're in can help break the mental loop.

(6) Practising self-care

Practising self-care is essential for managing these types of thoughts. Being kind to ourselves every day — not just on bad days — helps us build the skills needed to unlearn harmful cognitive distortions.

If this feels difficult or challenging, that's because it is. Unlearning cognitive distortions can take time. Even when we learn to recognise them, they can still affect us emotionally. Every time you catch yourself slipping into a distortion, write it down — dedicate a blank page in this book for them! There's plenty of material available on this topic, so read up, explore CBT models, and, if you're comfortable, speak to a therapist or trusted friend. Yes, this process can be tough, but it's possible to change these painful ways of thinking

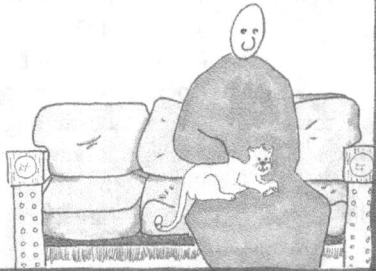

For A4 and printable versions of this worksheet, visit www.jeremysachs.com

Addictions and compulsions

The terms compulsive behaviour and addiction are often used interchangeably but they are different from one another. Many survivors will be familiar with one or both of them. Compulsive behaviours are 'repetitive behaviours that people feel compelled to engage in due to obsessions. These obsessions create a sense of anxiety, so people engage in compulsive behaviours to relieve those feelings of distress'.[4] They can cause us emotional distress when we act on them, even if they also bring some short-term mental relief. Generally, compulsive behaviours are intense and distracting urges to do something, which we either act on or do not. Compulsive behaviours can be common in survivors, for example compulsive sex, see Chapter 7, page 136.

Addiction is different. According to the American Society of Addiction Medicine, addiction is 'a chronic disease that involves compulsively using substances or engaging in behaviours that continue despite harmful consequences'.[5] Though this may seem similar to compulsive behaviour, in addiction, we are driven to consume something because it creates feelings of pleasure or euphoria, rather than being driven to do something to satisfy the urge. Both compulsive behaviour and addiction can be activated through distress or a desire to change from one emotional state to another, but generally speaking, compulsions are triggered by painful thoughts or feelings about ourselves or our world, while addictions can also be triggered by external factors, like exposure to similar addictive behaviour. You have likely seen films or TV where a recovering addict is knowingly or unknowingly offered a drink, reactivating their addiction.

Both addictions and compulsive behaviours are treatable. Compulsive behaviours may require CBT and/or medication, such as a selective serotonin reuptake inhibitor (SSRI). Addictions may require therapy, medication, and/or time to detox safely. You'll find signposting for resources at the end of this chapter (page 207).

Belief systems

When talking about something sensitive in the therapy room, I'll often say something like, 'I want to hold this idea delicately'. This phrase invites nuance and space to explore ideas that might have complicated stigma or harmful stereotypes or expectations associated with them. For many, religious faith can be such a topic. Religion is a divisive subject among survivors, especially male survivors. For survivors abused in a religious context or whose identity is commonly stigmatised by religious groups, the idea that religious faith might help with their trauma is impossible to believe, or even triggering (see Chapter 8, page 158 for more). However, for survivors who are religious or have strong faith in a belief system, faith can be a critical and connective part of their recovery. Some survivors may feel caught in the middle, with religious faith that is important to them but complicated by their identity, experience of abuse, or both. Such survivors' relationship with faith may leave them constantly questioning themselves and their place within their faith community. I am keen not to attack or label any belief system as an unsustainable coping strategy, but I do want to hold the idea of a belief system delicately. This is because some survivors may abandon themselves into a belief system in order to avoid the pain and confusion of abuse. This can come at the cost of other relationships or lead to further exploitation.

Belief systems that become unsustainable

Belief systems can work well as coping strategies. They can even replace the trauma lens in the short term because they help us make sense of the world, providing a guide for how to live and helping us cope with traumatic feelings or memories. Belief systems can include contemporary versions of stoicism, modern philosophy, spirituality, or religion, as well as self-help books written by public figures, positive psychology, radical politics, and conspiracy theories. They can vary widely, from helpful principles to harmful ideologies. Their appeal makes sense. When we have found ourselves the victim of senseless abuse, why wouldn't we want to find a coping strategy that makes sense of the world and helps us feel in control? Many belief systems are harmless, and investing in them can be a lifesaver, but for some survivors, they can make matters worse. Some men hold on to their belief systems so rigidly that an emotionally painful event, such as a relationship breakdown, bereavement, activated cPTSD, or job loss, can threaten the belief system and feel destabilising. In these cases, we may feel traumatised by the emotionally painful event, but the real trouble is that the belief system that helped us understand the world starts to become less effective, allowing the trauma lens to creep back in and taint the world.

Therapy can be challenging for both the therapist and the survivor whose belief system has been disrupted. Both want the survivor to feel better. A survivor may tell the therapist they want to finally explore their sexual trauma in order to be free from the aftermath of abuse. The therapist may agree to this, employing all their non-directive skills of listening, understanding, and gentle questioning, but soon, the therapy may start to feel stuck for both survivor and therapist. Perhaps the survivor is fighting to return to a time when his belief system worked for him, making him feel powerful and in control of his trauma systems. Meanwhile, the therapist may be trying to get the survivor to unpack the trauma he survived, returning to a time when he had little power. Both therapist and survivor may start to wonder why they are making so little progress, unaware that they are pulling the therapy in different directions. Therapy often ends fairly unceremoniously under these circumstances. The survivor may say they have benefited or made some breakthroughs, but either money or other commitments means the therapy needs to end. The therapist may be left feeling like they helped a little – perhaps even being available for the survivor when things were especially bad – but never really got to know the survivor or fully understand what they needed. After therapy ends, the client reestablishes a relationship with a potentially unsustainable belief system that makes them feel in control until the next event that disrupts their world view.

Desire for change is present even alongside unsustainable coping strategies. Even the most destructive behaviour may be a desperate attempt to shift from a distressing emotional state to one that feels better, even if 'better' is actually unhealthy or destructive. When living with the legacy of sexual abuse, survivors can develop deep relationships with our unsustainable coping strategies because they promise to alter our mood, even if only for a short time. We can compare coping strategies to tools in a toolbox. Sexual abuse and other adverse life experiences often leave us with very few tools. What's more, the tools we have might not do a good job of helping us in the long run. They may patch up the odd hole, but they are not enough to fix our biggest problems. Recovery from sexual abuse is not about throwing away the tools we have, but adding new tools to our toolbox. That way, when things get difficult, we have multiple – hopefully sustainable – tools, to try when coping.

10.3   The sustainable

My colleague Katherine Cox uses the metaphor of clinging to the side of a cliff when she describes coping strategies. Fingers bloody, wind and rain beating you down, you try to hold on to crumbling rocks. It's a life-or-death situation, and the last thing you need is someone offering you a kale smoothie. Yesterday, a kale smoothie might have been perfect for an energy boost, but today you need helicopters, ropes, specialised shoes, and a team of mountain goats to guide you to safety.

Katherine's metaphor illustrates that we need different coping strategies at different times and in different situations. On most days, a kale smoothie can sustain us, but during a crisis, we need more than just blended greens. Having multiple strategies available to help us cope means we stand a better chance of getting through difficult times – whether they last hours, days, weeks, months, or even years. A coping strategy that helped last week might not work this week, leaving us confused. In these moments, we need alternative strategies ASAP, which is one reason why this book includes a variety of coping exercises. They ensure that 1) you have plenty of options to try, and 2) even if one coping exercise doesn't work for you right now, it may be helpful in the future.

Coping strategies are another area of recovery impacted by survivors' identity or circumstances. Access to therapy illustrates this disparity well. Those who can afford it can seek regular counselling for as long as they need, in whatever modality they find most suitable. In contrast, in Britain, for example, survivors with lower incomes often have to rely on the NHS for counselling, which usually involves a waiting list for treatment that typically lasts six weeks and offers a limited range of therapeutic modalities. Additionally, therapists are underrepresented by people from minority backgrounds. In the British Association for Counsellors and Psychotherapists' (BACP) 2022–23 member survey, the majority of respondents (88.38 per cent) identified as white and between the ages of 45 and 65. While many white, older therapists are capable of working cross-culturally, this demographic imbalance may create an added burden for men from minority communities who must do the additional labour of seeking out a culturally sensitive therapist. This is important because we know according to studies that clients

> praised therapists who demonstrated culture-specific knowledge, skills in navigating racial/cultural dynamics inside and outside of therapy, and awareness of the importance of race and culture in shaping individual experience and identity and criticized those who displayed cultural ignorance or insensitivity.[6]

Survivors of any background can feel like we are alone in finding our way to heal, particularly men, who often believe they must deal with problems by themselves. It's tempting to believe that if we simply find that 'one thing' that helps – the right therapist, belief system, or coping strategy – everything else will make sense, and we'll heal. However, I don't believe it works this way. If there was one definitive way to heal from trauma, stress, and anxiety, there wouldn't be so many different books in the self-help section of any bookshop.

I believe we need to foster new connections in order to cope. This is why I run groups for survivors. While one-to-one therapy, self-help books, or individual coping strategies may be useful or even lifesaving, fostering new connections is a long-term, sustainable way to manage and reduce the impacts of sexual abuse. This process can be scary because it requires us to try new things, but if we want our brain to respond to the world differently than it did in the past, we need to expose it to new things. This is what connection is all about. It can look different to different people and can occur in a variety of environments, including online gaming communities, gardening or foraging groups, sports teams, hobby groups, charity volunteering, or support groups for survivors. All of these can help to soften the pain of our past trauma, either directly or indirectly.

It may be difficult to know where to start forming new connections, especially for men, who are often told we need to manage things by ourselves. To help, I have broken down some of the key elements to consider when attempting new connective experiences. Think about what they mean to you and how you might be able to implement them.

1. Proactivity

We need to seek out new experiences proactively. This can take work; often, hobbies or groups are not on our doorstep. Our networks, where we live, and our economic status all affect how easily we find new connections. Further, we might find a group of people who seem perfect on paper, but with whom we just don't gel in reality. This can be disheartening. We may feel like we're the odd ones out, when in truth, we just need to stick with it and find the next new opportunity for connection.

It can be hard when life gets busy to find proactive energy for something that may feel non-essential. However, finding new ways to connect in our lives is an essential and sustainable way of managing trauma.

2.   Relational experience

I know many people who describe their hobbies or interests as therapy: running, reading, listening to self-help talks, going on walks, or solo trips to the cinema. I know what they mean; all of these can be therapeutic and healthy. Many men enjoy these activities because they allow us to work on ourselves by ourselves. However, I argue that these are therapeutic, but not therapy. One key difference is that therapy is a relational experience with another person, and this is crucial for us as humans. A solo run may be wonderful for your mental health, but it isn't a relational experience. As humans, we need contact with other humans. We need to chat about the weather, debrief on the latest TV shows, and share stories. These relational experiences do not have to include serious or heavy conversations; you can just talk about *Love Island*, as long as you are having a pleasant experience with another human. Sure, this informal experience isn't therapy either, but I'd argue it is an essential ingredient to recovery that solo therapeutic activities can't give us.

Why, you might wonder, *would this sort of chit chat help me heal from trauma? I don't have time for that, and it doesn't sound important.* It all comes back to the trauma lens and how, as survivors, we can view everything, even the small things, through it. Practising low-stakes relational experiences can signal to our brain that *maybe* the trauma lens isn't the only way to view the world. If we can sustain relational experiences with acquaintances semi-regularly, we may start to see some of the cognitive distortions we carry with us as less true or powerful.

3.   Finding our experience reflected

Not so long ago, therapists believed that to heal from trauma, we needed to sit in a professional's office and tell our story. Telling our abuse story was treated as the finishing line in some therapeutic marathon, at the end of which survivors would finally be able to move on with their lives. We now know that this is not the case; in fact, pushing a survivor to talk about their trauma when they are not ready can be damaging and retraumatising.

Despite this, it can be powerful to share our stories. Telling another person the shameful, painful and dark parts of our lives can bring us a step closer to healing. Knowing that one other human in the world has heard what happened to us and not judged us is big, especially when we are used to locking emotions away or being the person everyone else relies on for support. We can achieve this by talking to a loved one or therapist about our experiences. These people may not have the same experience as us but still be able to listen without judgement. Or we could achieve this sharing in a survivor's group where other people have similar experiences to us. Being believed, respected, and not judged can be a big step toward recovery.

I do not believe anyone should be forced to tell their story. Sexual abuse is, among many things, a loss of control to someone else, which means that it is important for us to protect our boundaries. A therapist or healthcare professional who forces us to tell our stories is disregarding our boundaries. However, if you do want to share your story, I encourage you to do so (see Chapter 9, 'Disclosure', page 184, for tips on doing this).

4.   Gentleness with ourselves

For some men, even the words *gentleness with ourselves* can feel uncomfortable. You might already find yourself cringing, joking, or dismissing the idea. After all, modern Western masculinity often does not allow space for men to be gentle. It can demand that we be tough 100 per cent of the time. This is hard, and men may beat ourselves up for falling short of these impossible masculine ideals. We may compare ourselves to others or chastise ourselves for mistakes we feel we've made, and this can lead to depression, anxiety, or shame.

Being gentle with ourselves means working to accept that we are all on a journey through a process and no one moment defines us. We will mess up and behave in ways we wish we hadn't. We will have off days when we are unproductive or feel useless. Being gentle with ourselves means accepting that we are more than our actions on a bad day. In doing this, we allow ourselves to connect with the world, rather than allowing depression, anxiety or shame keep us isolated from it.

5.   Playfulness

Play comes naturally to almost all mammals; from tiger cubs to dolphins, we all have a sense of play. Humans are born with the ability to connect and play with those around us. As toddlers, we delight in games with our parents or carers, and at school, we form friendships often based on playfulness.

Adult humans often lose our ability to play somewhere along the way. For some, play is replaced by the self-consciousness of adolescence, followed by the responsibilities of adulthood. Playing in adulthood generally can feel daunting and vulnerable. Often, we don't know where to start or it feels like the demands of life don't allow us time to play. When we do get to play, it is often competitive and wrapped up in expressions of dominance and skill, rather than play for the sake of play. For some survivors, a sense of play is taken from us, sexual abuse robs us of the innocence required to play freely.

When I started running groups for male survivors, one of the many things that surprised me was the amount of laughter in each group. Each new group would get to a point when the members were comfortable enough to start playing, which included anything from funny stories about the day to dark humour about abuse that survivors could only enjoy within the group. Laughter became an essential part of the group process – so essential that I now encourage survivors to prioritise playfulness as much as therapy. Importantly, this playfulness needs to involve others, including people at a hobby or sports club, online games forum, or weekend socials. Playing is a huge part of connection. For survivors who were abused in childhood or grew up in an environment where we could not play, learning to play in adulthood is a bold and radical act of defiance against the abuse.

6.   Asking for support

Asking for support is often difficult for men. For many of us, it is so alien that simply finding the right words is a challenge. Further, some men may try asking for support but be denied it due to stigma, stereotypes, or identity. Many male survivors reach a point when we know we need help and summon the courage to approach a friend or support service, only to have our experience minimised, disbelieved, or ridiculed. When this is our experience, it is unlikely that we'll want to ask for help again.

Because you picked up this book, however, I know that part of you is looking for change. Like Rogers' potatoes on page 193, you are using everything within your reach to make sense of trauma and abuse. Challenge yourself to ask for support. You don't have to tell your abuse story to anyone, but practise reaching out. If you have an ache or pain that you keep meaning to see a doctor for, why not make an appointment? You can message a friend saying you feel down and want a catch-up. You can call an anonymous helpline when you feel anxious. Experiment with small acts of asking for support. If one doesn't work, be gentle with yourself and try another.

No one sustainable coping strategy can help everyone. No magic pill, philosophy, or therapeutic intervention can heal us all in one go. If we can accept we'll need different coping strategies at different times, offer ourselves gentleness, and foster connections, we will stand a better chance of managing our trauma. By connecting with the world, we can build a life after abuse and start to become the person we want to be. Building a toolkit of things that help us cope is a useful step towards this goal. For a guide on building a care plan, see chapter 12, page 240.

Urge surfing is a short-term technique we can use to avoid acting on urges we feel are harmful to us, such as smoking, overeating, online shopping, or substance use. This tool is used based on several factors:

- Urges rarely last longer than 30 minutes if we do not act on them, for example, by ruminating on, planning, justifying, or actually doing them.
- Sitting with our urges rather than trying to fight, distract from, or suppress them will eventually reduce the urge's power.
- Urges can feel all-encompassing, like they will never go away, but with practice, we can diminish them, and they can lose their power over us.

As you sit with your urge, imagine the wave, growing and getting stronger. Remind yourself that eventually, it will pass.[7]

Urge Surfing

③ PEAK

② RISE

④ FALL

① TRIGGER

Intensity of craving or urge

Length of time the craving or urge lasts

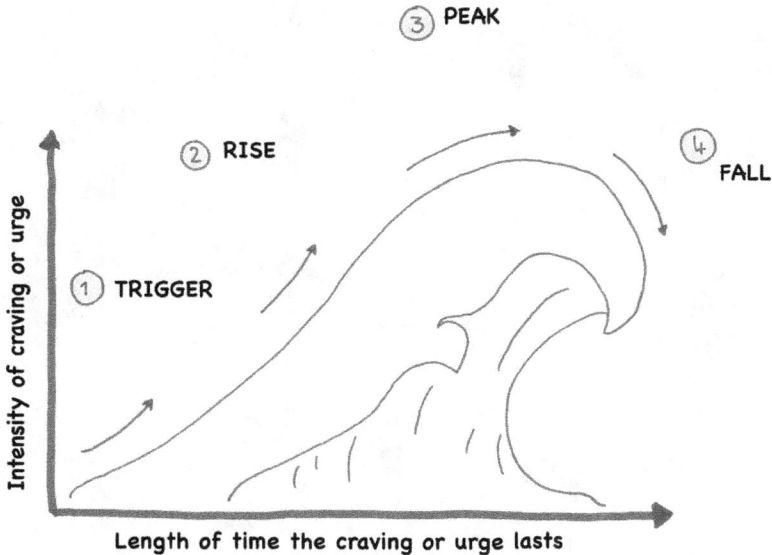

① TRIGGER: The urge is triggered by a situation, person or some thought or feeling.

② RISE: The urge becomes more intense. This can happen quickly or gradually.

③ PEAK: The urge is now at full strength and feels like it will never go away unless acted on.

④ FALL: The urge starts to lose it's intensity and eventually fades away.

Fighting urges often gives them more intensity and strength. Instead, try to simply notice your urges. Observe the physical sensations, focus on them, and describe what you feel. Pay attention to your breathing, or use breathing exercises. Some people visualise the urge becoming lighter with each breath. Remember, urges eventually pass, so allow them to fade naturally. This takes practice, so give yourself time to improve your skill in urge surfing.

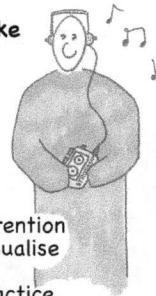

www.jeremysachs.com   @JeremySachs_

For A4 and printable versions of this worksheet, visit www.jeremysachs.com

For A4 and printable versions of this worksheet, visit www.jeremysachs.com

Resources

Shame (2011)

This film, directed by Steve McQueen, explores the life of a successful New Yorker grappling with his relationship with sex. As his addiction spirals out of control, he faces personal and professional consequences. This film is for adults and includes explicit scenes, so please watch with caution.

The Addicted Mind podcast

https://theaddictedmind.com/podcast/
In their own words, 'The Addicted Mind Podcast offers hope, understanding, and guidance for those dealing with addiction, with real stories and research to inspire and show the journey to recovery is worth it'.

Signposting

Action for Addiction

www.actiononaddiction.org.uk/partner-charities
Action on Addiction UK is a charity that focuses on providing treatment, prevention, and support for individuals affected by addiction, including substance abuse and behavioural dependencies. This website provides information on this and partner charities.

SMART Recovery UK

https://smartrecovery.org.uk
SMART Recovery offers support groups and online resources for individuals recovering from addiction to drugs, alcohol, and behaviours. Their programme is based on cognitive-behavioural techniques and self-empowerment principles.

Release

www.release.org.uk
Release provides human rights-focused legal advice, information, and support to individuals and families affected by drug addiction. They also advocate for drug policy reform and work to promote harm reduction approaches.

Addaction

www.wearewithyou.org.uk
Addaction offers a wide range of addiction treatment and support services across the UK. They provide support for individuals struggling with alcohol, drugs, and addictive behaviours, as well as support for families affected by addiction.

Notes

1   Carl R. Rogers, *A Way of Being* (Boston: Houghton Mifflin, 1995).
2   Regina J. Johnson, Michael W. Ross, Wendell C. Taylor, Mark L. Williams, Raul I. Carvajal, and Ronald J. Peters, 'Prevalence of childhood sexual abuse among incarcerated males in county jail', *Child Abuse and Neglect* 30, no. 1 (January 2006): 75–86, doi: 10.1016/j.chiabu.2005.08.013.
3   Kat Ford, Emma R. Barton, Annemarie Newbury, Karen Hughes, Zoe Bezecky, Janine Roderick, and Mark A. Bellis, 'Understanding the prevalence of adverse childhood experiences (ACEs) in a male offender population in Wales: The prisoner ace survey 2019', Public Health Wales NHS Trust, 2019. https://phw.nhs.wales/files/aces/the-prisoner-ace-survey, accessed 2 August 2024.
4   Judy Luigjes, Valentina Lorenzetti, Sanneke de Han, George J. Youssef, Carsten Murawski, Zsuzsika Sjoerds, et al., 'Defining compulsive behavior', *Neuropsychology Review* 29 (2019): 4–13.
5   'Definition of addiction', American Society of Addiction Medicine, 2024. www.asam.org/quality-care/definition-of-addiction, accessed 2 August 2024.
6   Doris F. Chang and Alexandra Berk, 'Making cross-racial therapy work: A phenomenological study of clients' experiences of cross-racial therapy', *Journal of Counseling Psychology* 56, no. 4 (October 2009): 521–536, doi: 10.1037/a0016905.
7   'Urge surfing', Dartmouth-Hitchcock, n.d. www.dartmouth-hitchcock.org/sites/default/files/2021-03/urge-surfing.pdf, accessed 2 August 2024.

Chapter 11

Moving forward with life

Chapter Contents

Finding my peace

When I began sharing my experience of abuse, many people offered advice on what they thought I should do. This is only natural; when someone you care about reveals something terrible, the instinct is to help. Because I've chosen to be vocal about my abuse, many people are aware, and as a result, I've received a lot of advice. Generally, people fall into two camps: those who believe I should report to the police and those who think I should forgive the perpetrator.

I'm now at a point where I'm comfortable discussing my choices and explaining why they're right for me. However, when I first started opening up, it was much more challenging. Although not intentional, the conversation often shifted to focus on the other person. After I disclosed my abuse, they would share their own trauma, suggest what had worked for them, or insist on therapies I 'needed' to try. Others reacted with anger or emotion, pressuring me to take the actions they believed were best, leaving me feeling overwhelmed.

I felt I had to manage their expectations about what I would do next. If I chose not to report the abuse, I feared disappointing them. If I did report it, I worried about betraying some social code because of distrust in the police. Similarly, if I didn't want to forgive, I sensed their disapproval, and if I mentioned considering forgiveness, they'd respond with, 'You're a better person than me; I could never...' – as if that was helpful.

DOI: 10.4324/9781003423331-11

For a time, this made me feel trapped. I hesitated to share with anyone, fearing it would be too burdensome. This strain made my relationships harder and, in turn, made it difficult for me to process and move on.

I'm in a place now where I am happy (a relative word) with the decisions I have made in order to feel a sense of peace about what happened to me. When I disclose to people, I am clear why I decided to do what I did and how it has helped me process the pain of sexual abuse. Occasionally, I have to be really clear that I'm not interested in hypotheticals or answering questions from people that feel energy sapping. It is something that happened to me in my past and while I can talk about it now, I'm much more interested in talking about my future.

Anonymous

Many sexual abuse survivors ask themselves a version of the question, 'When do I get to put abuse behind me and move on with my life?' This question makes a lot of sense. When something so painful and unfair happens to us, we can desperately want to heal in order to get on with our lives. It can feel like sexual abuse has held us back for years, sometimes decades. Abuse can make us feel like we have been robbed of opportunities and a chance for success. Now, after so much struggle, we want a 'normal' life like so many people around us appear to have.

There are plenty of reasons survivors may struggle to move forward. Some may find their abuser continues to have power over them, even years after the abuse ends. This may be especially complicated when the perpetrator is a family member or other member of the survivor's social circle or a celebrity or public figure. Under these circumstances, the consequences of disclosing can feel so life-altering to survivors and those around us, that they stop us from feeling like we can come forward. This can make survivors feel that we are even more powerless and our perpetrators even more powerful. It can feel like we may never escape the shadow of abuse. For example, over a 50-year period, British TV personality Jimmy Savile was reported to have abused approximately 500 men, women, boys, and girls. He did this in hospitals, including children's hospitals, as well as the BBC broadcasting studios. He died in 2011, and survivors began coming forward in 2012. Savile had power over not only his victims but also those who ignored his actions, consciously or unconsciously allowing the abuse to happen. It was only after his death that survivors felt his power over them break, allowing some to feel safe enough to disclose the abuse in order to move forward. Male survivors often attempt to break abusers' power and move on by reporting them and seeking a criminal conviction. However, as we discussed in Chapter 9 ('Disclosure', see page 173), the journey from reporting to conviction can be fraught, placing further strain on survivors through a criminal justice system in need of reform.

In this chapter, I want to acknowledge that moving forward typically involves finding some sort of inner peace and that criminal prosecution and forgiveness are often held up as the two main solutions available to men. However, neither solution is as straightforward as many people believe, and the hope that they will 'fix things' or 'let that be the end of it' rarely plays out in reality, particularly for men's emotional healing. I will also introduce the concept of transformative justice, a political framework created by and for minoritised communities (eg, Indigenous, Black, immigrant, and LGBTQIA+ communities, communities of colour, poor and low-income communities, people with disabilities, sex workers) responding to violence, harm, and abuse.[1] My aim is not to suggest that you must choose one way or another to move forward but to provide you with information and tools you may wish to use to explore your own relationship to forgiveness, justice, and moving forward. In my experience, survivors' relationship with abuse and abusers can change over time, which means we need new ways to make sense of the abuse's aftermath. Hopefully, this chapter will give you some new ideas about going forward in your life.

11.1   Forgiveness

Forgiveness is a big topic, and not just for survivors. It has meant different things depending on cultural, religious, or philosophical beliefs throughout history. While it is a universal idea, it is also abstract, with no one fixed definition. It will look or feel different depending on who we speak to. Forgiveness may come from individuals or communities who have been wronged, harmed, or oppressed. Individuals and, indeed, whole states may ask for forgiveness or apologise for wrongs done: in July 2023, for example, Willem-Alexander, King of the Netherlands, apologised for his ancestors' role in the colonial slave trade. However, as survivors, we often think of forgiveness as an individual act. Across the Abrahamic religions, when someone does something bad, they must repent to be forgiven by God. Those of us who were not raised in a religious setting have no doubt also learned about forgiveness. Soap operas, reality TV programmes, and films all create narratives about forgiveness, but these narratives can be contradictory. Some suggest that forgiveness is necessary, while others focus on retribution instead. Many men internalise these contradictory views. We may understand that forgiveness is largely considered a good thing while also feeling that simple forgiveness is weak, allowing someone else to walk all over us.

Among survivors of sexual abuse, forgiveness can be a polarising issue. Some men believe forgiveness is a powerful tool necessary to heal from sexual abuse, while others fantasise about violent revenge against their abusers. Still others say they wish to work towards forgiving their abuser but are not ready to do so. Some men still know their abuser and do not want to think about forgiveness until they are separated from the abuser or the abuser dies. When deciding whether or not to forgive abusers, survivors can feel influenced by many opinions, which can be confusing. Ultimately, however, the meaning of *forgiveness* will be unique to each survivor's personal beliefs, experiences and culture. Forgiveness is a decision you need to make for yourself, and no one has a right to tell you whether or how to forgive.

What forgiveness means to you

Many external factors can influence whether we forgive or not. If we experience abuse as a child or adolescent that is perpetrated by a family member or someone close to the family, survivors may feel pressure to forgive from our family. This can be disturbing, as if our forgiveness is what our family needs to move on from the abuse. It can feel like the people who are meant to support us want the whole thing to go away, and the sooner we forgive, the sooner they can put it behind them. Some may see our forgiveness as a signal that they don't have to deal with our abuse and can ignore the harm done to us. Sometimes perpetrators themselves put pressure on survivors to forgive 'for the sake of the family' or guilt us into forgiveness by saying things like, 'If you don't get over it, you'll be hurting people you love'.

In some cultures, forgiveness is framed as a religious issue. For devout survivors, this focus on forgiveness can be so prominent that our personal feelings are pushed aside and replaced with our community's religious beliefs. Loved ones may tell us, 'God wants us to forgive' or, 'I will pray that you gain the strength to forgive'. Though religious frameworks can offer structure that can be an additional source of support, they also have the potential to push survivors towards forgiveness before they are ready. They may even be used by family members or the wider community to minimise abuse. Whether the abuse occurs within or outside a religious community, some families or communities may use religious faith to apply additional pressure on survivors to move on. Framing forgiveness in a purely religious context or as evidence of survivors' faith can deny us the opportunity to fully explore our feelings towards the perpetrator and their actions. It can also undermine survivors' ability to fully trust our family or community members, making us feel that their support or love is conditional on our forgiveness. Within this framework it might feel that the family unit or community is being prioritised over the experience of the individual in a way that might feel selfish or even malicious. However, sexual abuse can be not only upsetting but scary for survivors' families and religious communities, as their worlds may also be turned upside down. Some members may not want to think about it because the consequences are too terrible to imagine. Some may feel guilty for not protecting us, worry what others will think, or struggle to reconcile their own role, direct or otherwise, in the abuse.

For many survivors, religious faith or practice can be helpful and healing. Religion can provide a physical, spiritual, or mental space, away from everyday life, that allows us to decide how we feel about the harm done to us and whether or not we want to forgive. It is important, however, that any decision we make to forgive in a religious context is wholly our own, not the result of pressure by a belief system that tells us forgiveness is obligatory. Forgiving an abuser because our religion tells us it's compulsory can provide comfort for a while, but, much like the belief systems we discussed in Chapter 10 ('Coping,' page 198), religion can become an unsustainable coping strategy if it allows us never to deal with the pain of abuse.

In some instances, forgiveness can become a burdensome finishing line, an obligatory endpoint we're supposed to strive for. It can occupy all of our energy, because: 1) if we focus on forgiveness, we can avoid sitting with the pain of what happened to us; and 2) other people can convince us that forgiveness is the only way to feel better. Even therapists can get caught in this way of thinking. In my early days as a charity worker working with male survivors, there was a tendency during sessions, whether conscious or not, to veer towards talking about forgiveness. Rather than delving into the profound anguish, shame, and betrayal stemming from their experiences of sexual abuse, clients and I often shifted focus towards more comfortable questions like, 'Do you wish to forgive?', followed by discussions about forgiveness. The survivor and I both would unconsciously conspire to steer discussions towards forgiveness and relief, and away from processing the pain.

Whether you want to forgive or not, it helps to think of forgiveness as something we need to continuously work on, rather than a finishing line. I have worked with men who felt for decades that they had been able to forgive their perpetrator but then learned some new information or a long-buried memory surfaced that tested, or even retracted, their forgiveness. Such new information may be the final straw for some survivors, who may no longer want to spend energy forgiving someone who harmed them. As we grow and learn new things about ourselves, our relationship to forgiveness can change too. For some survivors, this may mean finding alternative language to the word *forgiveness*.

11.2   Moving forward

Forgiveness is a word that implies a relationship with a perpetrator. It requires that we to face the perpetrator, either literally or symbolically, acknowledge what they did to us and offer our forgiveness for them to take, again, either literally or symbolically. For some survivors, this is too difficult. The damage was too profound, the betrayal too strong, and we do not want to offer anything to the perpetrator. In these cases, it can help to change our language. Rather than saying, 'I forgive', we can say, 'I am moving forward'. This change in language is significant. Unlike *forgiveness*, which implies we have a relationship with the perpetrator, the term *moving forward* focuses on our relationship to trauma and our hopes for the future. It orientates the process around survivors and our relationship with ourselves, rather than on the perpetrator. To move forward is to acknowledge the pain of our past without letting it influence our future.

Whether you want to find forgiveness or move forward, there are three areas I encourage survivors to address:

1. Letting go of our guilt and shame towards our own actions
2. Forgiving our harm to ourselves
3. Acknowledging our harm to others

1. Letting go of our guilt and shame towards our own actions

One of the toughest things we can do as survivors is sit with the guilt of what happened to us. As men, we may blame our adult or childhood selves for not defending ourselves or telling anyone, even if we know it was impossible. We may feel shame for our unsustainable coping strategies (eg, drinking too much) or for staying too long in abusive relationships. We may wonder why we made choices that appear counterintuitive to the goal of keeping ourselves safe. We may ask ourselves questions like,

- Why did I stay in that relationship so long?
- Why did I instigate sex with someone I knew was abusive (or had abused me previously)?
- Why did I go home with my abuser?
- Why do I still care about my abuser?
- Why did I think I could change my abuser if I stayed in the relationship?
- Should I have done something to stop it, even though I was a child?

Abusers may use their power over us not just in moments of sexual abuse but also more broadly. Their power over us can impact all aspects of our lives and make us do things that confuse and shame us when we look back on them.

In the following example, survivor Jules explains how the abuse he experienced held such power over him that he acted in ways that made him even more vulnerable to abuse. His story illustrates the power his abuser had over him, even when they weren't together. Ultimately, it demonstrates that sexual abuse isn't just an act or pattern of sexual violence, but also an insidious attempt to control and manipulate multiple aspects of a victim's life (locations and social media platforms have been removed from original testimony):

A part of me knew it was wrong, but I don't think that's how I thought of it then. I knew it was a secret, and I felt part excitement and part awfulness about it. I was in year 11 [ages 15–16] and was really quiet, especially for a boy in my school. I was stressed about exams when the geography teacher, Mr. Adams,[2] asked me to stay behind to look at my coursework. I didn't mind because I had nowhere else to be. This became a regular thing. Every Tuesday, I could go to his classroom, and he'd help me, or ask me about my future. I really liked someone taking an interest.

One day, the abuse started. He touched me on top of my trousers and was touching himself at the same time underneath his trousers. I didn't like it very much. I was scared of someone walking in and scared he would reject me if I moved or said no, so I froze. I just let him do it. I went back next Tuesday, hoping it was a one-off, but he did it again, and the pattern started. He did more things, and it all escalated each time until I left school.

A few years after college, he found me on social media and sent me a message. We started chatting, and after a month or so of chat, he invited me to go stay with him at a national park for the weekend. I got the train, and he picked me up and took me to a hotel room. When we went inside... I started to panic. It came out of nowhere. I felt trapped in the room with him, like I couldn't escape. I froze again. I had to stay the night. It was horrible; I was in pain, but he didn't notice. I eventually fell asleep.

The next morning, I cried. I think I was having a panic attack. He was telling me he hadn't done anything wrong, and I should just calm down. He refused to drive me to the train station, telling me I was being overly sensitive, and [he] told me I was an adult and could make my own way if I wanted to leave. I had to wait for two buses to go back to the train station. I hadn't showered and was still shaken up. I feel so much shame about the time at school, but it's crazy I went to meet him. I thought, *What's wrong with me? I must have wanted to do this, and it wasn't really abuse because I let it happen. I got on that train to meet* him*!*
—Jules, 38, straight, white

This story gives us a real sense of how Jules needed connection with another person and how his abuser took advantage of that to manipulate Jules into acting in the way he did. It's easy to see how Jules felt 'crazy' and ashamed when he looked back and tried to understand these actions. Many survivors have similar stories, in which their behaviour seemed to condone or seek out the abuse. These experiences can be deeply troubling for survivors, exacerbated by society's tendency to misinterpret this behaviour as consent. Ultimately, the responsibility for any act of abuse lies squarely with the perpetrator. It's crucial to recognise that abusers' influence extends far beyond the confines of the abuse itself, extending into the realm of control over victims' decisions and behaviours. Survivors must come to terms with the fact that the actions we took that caused us harm were the results of manipulation and coercion by individuals who disregarded our autonomy and right to consent, regardless of any deceptive rhetoric they may have employed. It can take us a long time to put the blame for such actions where it belongs: on the perpetrator.

2. Forgiving our harm to ourselves

In the last chapter we looked at some of the ways harming ourselves can result from a desire to cope with the pain of trauma. However, self-harm can also be passive, keeping us isolated or feeling stuck. Passive self-harm may not be the typical method people imagine men using to harm ourselves, but it can affect all parts of our lives: we may avoid relationships, stay in the same job, or feel that we have not lived up to our potential. Over time, fear of retraumatisation can damage our sense of worth and prevent us finding motivation to seek out ways to heal, leading to isolation. In the first episode of my podcast *The Trauma Talks*, I interviewed psychologist and author Dr Christiane Sanderson. According to Sanderson, when sexual abuse teaches us that 'relationships are dangerous, to stay away, this makes it hard to form the very types of relationships that could be healing, and that leads to incredible loneliness – what I call *traumatic loneliness*'.[3]

This *traumatic loneliness* can manifest as a form of self-neglect, in which we don't look after ourselves, nurture positive relationships or have life goals. We may wrap ourselves up in the mundane and predictable, insulating ourselves from potential trauma as well as from tools or methods of healing and preventing ourselves from moving on. Other survivors may harm ourselves through external means, such as alcohol, drugs, nicotine, or poor dietary choices. These forms of harm seldom impact us in isolation. They can also hurt the people around us – family members, work colleagues, or friends who care for us. In forgiving ourselves for self-neglect or destructive lifestyle choices, we can become able to acknowledge that we are doing the best we can with what we have.

3. Acknowledging our harm to others

It can be difficult accepting that we have harmed others, either inadvertently or deliberately, particularly when we are working to move on from harm done to us. It can be a painful truth to acknowledge that, because we were hurt by the experience of sexual abuse, we may have hurt others. Men, in particular, can find it challenging to talk about harm we have caused, and this often leads us to a shameful place that we may feel there is no coming back from. For many men, the mix of sexual abuse and a lack of safe space for men to talk about our feelings, leads to difficult emotions coming out in all sorts of problematic ways.

Often, we cause inadvertent harm through our behaviours. When we cheat on a partner, use substances or seek to harm ourselves, it often impacts those around us. Take an affair, for example. Even if we are never caught cheating on our partners, cheating can still do inadvertent harm to the relationship. A lack of intimacy or sex in the relationship can affect our partners, making them feel unattractive or that they have done something wrong. Our shame over having affairs might make us irritable to be around. Time invested in searching for sex outside of our relationship can put a strain on families. Survivors experiencing addiction to alcohol, a depressant drug, may see reduced quality in our emotional connection to our children. Though this is not be actively harmful to the child in the same way as physical or sexual abuse, these children may grow up feeling like we aren't fully available to them. They may become unsure of their own sense of worth or learn to mistrust affection.

Some survivors may actively harm people around them. They may become aggressive, argumentative, or abusive. For many survivors, toxic masculinity and sexual abuse block opportunities to develop ways of coping with the world that aren't harmful. When men project violence into the world, they are often giving us insight into their experiences or inner life. This doesn't make their behaviour acceptable, but admitting that we have done wrong and acknowledging that our aggression is a product of the violence we have faced can give survivors whose behaviour is harmful to others a useful starting point for change.

Coming to terms with the harm we have survived and the harm we have caused can feel daunting. You may have felt ashamed simply reading this section. Confronting painful and shaming events in our lives requires that we be as vulnerable and honest as possible. We may feel like we deserve extreme punishments or punish ourselves through destructive behaviours. While we need to be accountable, we need to achieve this without overly punishing ourselves. We can view the harm we cause as a symptom of our traumatic experience of sexual abuse, in the same way we might view nightmares or flashbacks. When we seek to forgive ourselves and move on, we are already beating our odds as survivors.

11.3   Transformative justice (TJ)

TJ is a political framework that seeks to respond to and end violence, harm, and abuse. Some of the earliest articulations of TJ principles can be found in the work of Black feminist scholars and activists such as Angela Davis, who critiqued the racism and inequities inherent in the criminal justice system.[4] However, TJ methods and ideas can be found throughout history, for example, within various Native American tribes that practised peace-making circles as a form of conflict resolution and healing. These circles brought together community members – including offenders, victims, and elders – to discuss harm and work towards healing and reconciliation.[5] Organisations like INCITE! Women of Color Against Violence and Critical Resistance,[6] founded in 2000, promote TJ frameworks as alternatives to the punitive approach of the criminal legal system. TJ frameworks emphasise community-based responses to harm, focusing on centring the needs of survivors, addressing root causes, and promoting healing and accountability.[7]

TJ exists outside of statutory systems, where violence not only commonly occurs, but is perpetuated, such as the criminal justice, health services, and asylum systems. People coming in contact with these statutory systems, who, in many cases, have been previously traumatised by similar institutions, may experience additional abuse and trauma. This trauma then perpetuates more violence within society. TJ interventions do not rely on the criminal justice system for justice, nor do they seek more violence – in other words, they do not involve 'eye-for-an-eye' justice, revenge, or vigilantism. Instead, TJ seeks to cultivate healing, harm reduction, safer communities, and importantly, accountability. I have asserted that sexual abuse does not occur in a vacuum; TJ is based around the idea that neither does violence. Poverty, insecure housing, war and displacement, white supremacy, capitalism, patriarchy, toxic masculinity, and misogyny all create an environment that cultivates violence and perpetuates it for future generations.

TJ as an alternative to the criminal justice system

I've been privileged to work with male survivors from many backgrounds and with many identities. Due to the diversity of my clients, I've seen many different types of experiences with the criminal justice system. Among the few survivors I have known who have taken their perpetrator to court and successfully won a case against them, I have noticed mixed feelings afterwards. Initially, they may have a sense of catharsis, relief that the legal process (which can last years) has finally come to an end, satisfaction that the perpetrator hasn't got away with it, or a sense of resolution. As the weeks and months go by, many survivors feel a return to normal – but as we know, 'normal' for survivors can be difficult. Their traumatic symptoms continue, and relationships are still a challenge. I have known men in the United States who were awarded thousands of dollars in compensation for their abuse but had not been able to spend it because they feel that it will allow the world to forget about them and their experience. I have known survivors who felt deeply disturbed and shamed when their perpetrators were named and shamed in local newspapers. Few male survivors, it seems, derive the kind of *straightforward* peace assumed with a successful legal procedure.

For many survivors, the burden of the criminal justice system is too much. An end-to-end review of rape cases conducted by the UK government found that 57 per cent of survivors who reported to the police in England and Wales in 2021/22 withdrew their case.[8] The reasons for this are multifaceted, but they include the length of time cases take, invasiveness and disruption that can exacerbate trauma, minority stress, and stigma. Some survivors simply don't trust the police to handle their experiences or trust the courts to be sensitive to the complexities that can come with rape and sexual abuse cases. Operation Soteria is a UK Home Office-funded research and change programme aimed at transforming the way police investigate rape and serious sexual violence. The programme's Year One report, published in December 2022, found that officers lacked specialist knowledge and 'demonstrated explicit victim blaming and lack of belief in the victim, which impacted on the subsequent investigation'. The report continues:

> Some [officers] stated that they believed that most reports of rape are just examples of 'regretful sex', or that if victims presented additional issues, such as mental health problems or alcohol/substance misuse, then this was the victim's problem and the legal system was not obligated to safeguard them.[9]

It is absolutely the case that some men have positive experiences with the police and the courts. If you are considering exploring criminal or civil justice, do not discount those options on the word of this book alone. However, because many survivors experience negative interactions with the criminal justice system, it's important that this book includes discussion about rethinking the meaning of *justice*.

Accessing TJ

Beginning to learn about TJ can become overwhelming. In addition to violence, TJ concerns the climate crisis, disability justice, land and housing ownership, criminal justice and healthcare, colonialism, and of course, sexual abuse. In some cases, TJ encourages survivors and perpetrators to work together towards accountability and healing. At the end of this chapter, I've included a link to the documentary *Hollow Water*, about a community of Indigenous Ojibway people in Canada who experienced an epidemic of sexual abuse, along with alcoholism, addiction, and suicide. The documentarians recorded survivors and perpetrators who convened in a 'community healing and sentencing circle' to create accountability and work towards ending the cycle of generational abuse.

It may feel benefitting from TJ requires that we first embrace radical politics, face our perpetrator, and take to the streets demonstrating against social injustice. Some survivors do these things, and that's great, but it's not for everyone. TJ can also be quiet, subtle, and very personal. Many survivors embrace TJ principles without knowing it. For example, I didn't realise my male survivor groups for SurvivorsUK used many TJ principles until I had been running them for some time. This is a common experience within TJ circles. Many facilitators, therapists, and community healers develop survivor services or safe spaces only to realise years later that there is a framework for the work they have been doing. Over the years, my survivor groups have developed alongside my understanding of TJ. This has given me time to think about which principles of TJ best apply to male survivors, either in the context of group, individual, or one-to-one practice. Some of these practices may not feel important to you right now, and that is okay. This is not a step-by-step healing guide, but a set of suggestions that may or may not feel currently tenable or useful in your recovery. Either is okay.

Five principles of TJ for survivors

1.   Dedicate time to what you love, preferably without monetisation

In therapy, it's common to hear people talk about 'doing the work'. For some, *doing the work* means facing your pain – turning up and having hard conversations. This mindset can appeal to men in particular. Often, we want to rip off the plaster, getting all the pain out in one intense action. We say to ourselves, *If I could do a week-long course of painful intense therapy, training, or trauma life coaching and get it over with, that would be the ideal way to move on.* Unfortunately, it is rare to heal from sexual trauma this way.

As an alternative, I suggest thinking about what you love. This may be a hobby, sport, or other activity, even something you once enjoyed and stopped doing for some reason. Reconnect with that activity, pour time into it, take it seriously and prioritise it in the same way you might prioritise work, the gym, or a family responsibility. Build it into your weekly schedule and find ways to engage with it depending on the time you have. For example, if you decide you're going to dedicate time to foraging mushrooms, set a date in your diary to spend a day in parks or woods looking for them. If you don't have a schedule that allows weekly trips to the local woods, you may look for other ways to engage, as well. This could include reading about mushrooms, buying a home grow kit, or joining social groups centred on mushrooms, either in person or online. Whether mushroom-related or not, ring-fence time in your week to nurture what you love to do.

I often insist men choose an activity without attempting to monetise it. I do this because in recent decades, people seem to increasingly prioritise hobbies that can in some way generate capital. Suddenly, activities we once did just for ourselves need to become a 'side hustle'. Instead of just painting, for example, we may feel pressure to set up an online shop where we sell our paintings or to use social media to gain attention and 'likes' for them. Capitalising on our hobbies can quickly take away the joy and pleasure we feel engaging with what we love. Our enjoyment soon becomes enmeshed with other people's validation, and the goal shifts from doing something because we love to do it to doing it for likes, external validation, or money.

If you create or do something you're proud of, by all means, share it with loved ones. If someone wants to give you money for something you produce through your hobby, go ahead and accept if you want to. But make sure your relationship with your hobby doesn't become linked to other people's value of it, creating competitiveness and external and internal judgement that can destroy your joy in what you love.

2. Let go of chastising and bitter mindsets

Many survivors know what it is like to sit with punishing, angry feelings, wanting to punish our perpetrators and ourselves. We may have fantasies of violence or destruction that can be indiscriminate, projected onto strangers, loved ones, perpetrators, and ourselves. Many of us feel bitter that other people had opportunities we didn't because sexual abuse held us back and kept us trapped. In many ways, we *need* to feel like this. It may feel like raging against what has been done to us is what keeps us from losing ourselves to despair or fading into annihilation. However, rage can only help us for so long before it turns our whole world grey and bitter and we start to chastise everyone around us for any wrong they do or success they achieve. The pain of abuse can bleed into our world view, keeping us isolated. For those of us from a minoritised community, this can be particularly acute. Both the experiences of abuse and othering can keep us feeling like we are on the outside looking in. The temptation to sink into a chastising and bitter mindset can be powerful.

Breaking this mindset can be hard, but it is necessary if we want to change our lives. While the social oppression or stigma we face is out of our control, we can make decisions about our own thought patterns. We can choose not to interpret other people's successes as personal wounds to us or rely on self-deprecating humour (something I still struggle with). If we catch ourselves chastising others or ourselves, we can consciously notice it and move on rather than allowing that feeling to fester.

3. Acknowledge systemic violence and reject capitalism

Sexual abuse is a deeply personal trauma that can haunt survivors for years or decades after it ends. It can be challenging to step back and see the ways in which Western society perpetuates sexual abuse. Despite the challenge, understanding this context is important for preventing future abuse and understanding how to move forward. Throughout this book, I give examples of ways in which society silences survivors and creates conditions that protect abusers, including toxic masculinity that ignores male survivors, stigma and myths that spread harmful misinformation about survivors, sexual stereotypes that blame victims, and statutory institutions that harm survivors rather than help. All of these examples contribute to *systemic violence*, which is the harm people suffer from social structures, including social and statutory institutions that sustain and create harm. Systemic violence results from the inequalities on which Western society was founded and which still affect its members today, including male survivors. These inequalities not only make it harder for survivors to get help, but they also protect perpetrators by creating environments in which they can victimise vulnerable people.

TJ aims to combat these cycles of systemic violence in both collective and individual ways. One step individuals can take is rejecting certain forms of capitalism. This claim sometimes invites some very sceptical looks and raised eyebrows. People become suspicious that I'm about to ask them to give up their jobs and worldly belongings for life on a commune in the rural countryside. Rather than resorting to that extreme, however, I encourage survivors to consider how they engage with some forms of capitalism. So much of our Western society relies on our feeling inadequate or that we need to change to fit into a narrow definition of manhood. Capitalism deliberately fuels these feelings of inadequacy because it directly benefits from them, selling us solutions and quick fixes, everything from crash diets and one-size-fits-all life coaching to food and clothing. This is harmful for most people, in my experience; however, it can be especially harmful for survivors, who often already feel inadequate due to the abuse. Anything that sustains stringent ideas of how men should be – strong, young, non-disabled, emotionally independent – silences male survivors by upholding myths and stigma about men and male survivors.

As an exercise, pay attention to how you feel next time you see an advert for an online fashion brand, gym supplement, diet or life coaching programme. Many brands deliberately attempt to make us feel bad in order to sell us their products. They may use muscled or skinny models or people who look happy or wealthy while using their products. They may tell us we 'need' what they are selling to be successful. Next time you see an advertisement like this, ask yourself, *Who is getting rich off making me feel bad about myself?*

Social media is another tool of capitalism that may affect us poorly. Social media platforms can be a tool for connectivity, and many survivors find support and like-minded individuals using them. However, they can also have harmful effects on us. Platforms use algorithms designed to keep us using them to generate advertising revenue. This can lead us to spend hours on social media, spread misinformation, and increase polarisation between groups. We may find ourselves in corners of the internet that fuel the dark or negative parts of our psyches. If we feel inadequate, as many survivors do, social media engagement often reinforces this.

Capitalist environments – particularly social media and advertising – may not directly create the circumstances where men are sexually abused, but they often reinforce stereotypes and promote toxic masculinity, tell us to spend money to solve psychological pain, and fuel negative outlooks that can become barriers to survivors getting support or being believed. In addition, they can keep us imprisoned in negative thought patterns about ourselves or the world. Disengaging from social media can give our minds a break from being bombarded with messages that make us feel bad and promote toxic masculinity and stigma about survivors.

4.   Find spaces where you can share yourself and your identity

One reason I advocate for group therapy is that sexual abuse causes us to hide so much of ourselves. Due to shame and social pressures, many men hide and repress much of our inner world. In group therapy, we can practise bringing our shameful thoughts and dark feelings to the surface. Often, we find that when we share our thoughts and feelings, other men are able to say, 'Me too!', and the heaviness of these dark thoughts and feelings starts to get lighter.

This isn't exclusive to group therapy. Groups focused on hobbies or interests can have similar effects. What is important, however, is that you feel able to bring your experiences and identity to the group. Joining any book club might be fun, but a gay man who joins an LGBTQIA+ book club has an opportunity not only to connect over a love of books but to see his identity reflected back to him in the other members. This can have a remarkable, powerful effect on survivors. Even if we aren't able to talk about the abuse, finding a space that reflects our interests and identity can be a big step towards healing. Further, having a group or individuals within a group with whom you feel you can share your identity may bring you a step closer to disclosing your experience to someone. Though I do not believe disclosing is something survivors *need* to do, I *do* believe in the healing benefit of having another person hear and believe your story, whether they are a friend, therapist, or members of a survivor group.

It may feel hard to prioritise finding groups like this, particularly in the modern world. The responsibilities of work and family can leave us with little or no time to find new spaces. However, whether they occur in group therapy for survivors or special interest groups for people who share your identity, group connections invite something new and positive into our life based around our interests, experiences, or identity and can help us move forward.

5. Make it a practice and make it individual

All of the principles and coping strategies in this book require that we practise them in our life. This may be one of the hardest parts of using TJ principles to move on because we must be brave and proactive and practise self-care. Recovery is seldom linear, and all survivors sometimes slip back into ways of being that harm us or make us feel bad. Embedding these principles into our daily practice gives us a good chance to move forward and experience positive change. Regularly reviewing our needs also allows us to make changes, because what we need today may not be what we need in the future. See Chapter 12, page 240 for how to build a personal care plan.

Another challenge is that each individual survivor must build their own practice in different ways. I can't tell you which therapy will work best for you or which hobbies or interests you should pursue. I can't tell you how many minutes on social media are too much for you or which spaces will be best to share your identity. These five principles make up a process of trial and error that will be different for each individual survivor. You will need to be proactive in your recovery by exposing yourself to new people and experiences. Ultimately, this is one of the strongest antidotes to the pain of sexual trauma, made more difficult because sexual abuse often results in survivors actively wanting to avoid proactiveness. Shame wants you to stay alone in the dark. Self-loathing wants to stop you trying new things. Trauma wants to keep you trapped in a dangerous world. The trauma of sexual abuse fights to keep you isolated, making it hard to move forward without proactive practice and trial and error. There is no one-size-fits-all approach to putting these principles into practice. Cultivating a proactive practice can be challenging, and it is important to treat yourself as kindly as possible while you do it. If you have a bad day, don't punish yourself for it; just allow yourself to draw a line underneath the day and start again the next. Remember it is unrealistic for men to expect to be our best selves every single day. I suspect it's an expectation fuelled (if not created) by capitalism and toxic masculinity to keep us making money for others. You are allowed off days, weeks, or months, as long as you recognise them and return to your practice of self-care.

Narrative Exposure Therapy (NET) is a short-term therapy developed to treat traumatic stress disorders. In this worksheet, I've borrowed a part of the NET process: creating a timeline of your life marked by specific key moments.

Creating one of these can be especially helpful if you struggle to remember your childhood or want to make sense of events that have shaped your life. It can also be a valuable tool for communicating to others the situations and environments you've lived through. Start by either drawing a string or use a real piece. Along the string, place these four objects to symbolise different important events in your life. Try and place them in as close to chronological order as possible.

The objects symbolise:

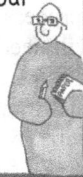

Stones: They symbolise the traumas we have survived in our past.

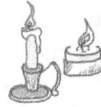

Candles: They symbolise losses, like relationships ending, divorce, bereavements or moving away from support networks.

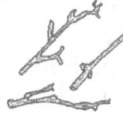

Sticks: They symbolise difficult things we've survived or done - not traumatic but certainly impactful.

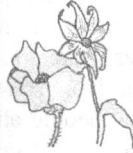

Flowers: They symbolise the good, positive, and joyful things we've experienced.

Often, the string begins at birth, but if you want to include intergenerational trauma or a family story, like migration, you can extend it further back. The end of the string is coiled to represent the life that remains. Here's an example I've created to show what one might look like:

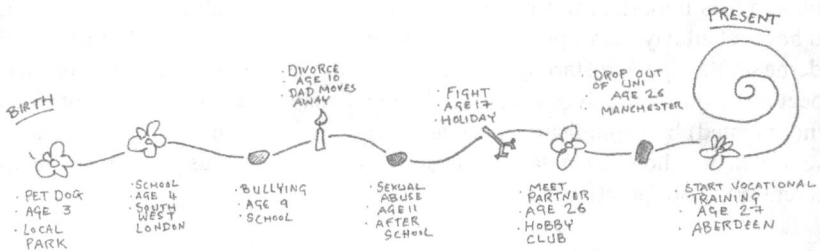

Label each symbol with a short title, for example, **Pet Dog**, then the age you were, **Age 3,** and finally where you were, **Local Park.**

Use this when you want to take time to think about your past and how it may impact you today.

www.jeremysachs.com   @JeremySachs_

For A4 and printable versions of this worksheet, visit www.jeremysachs.com

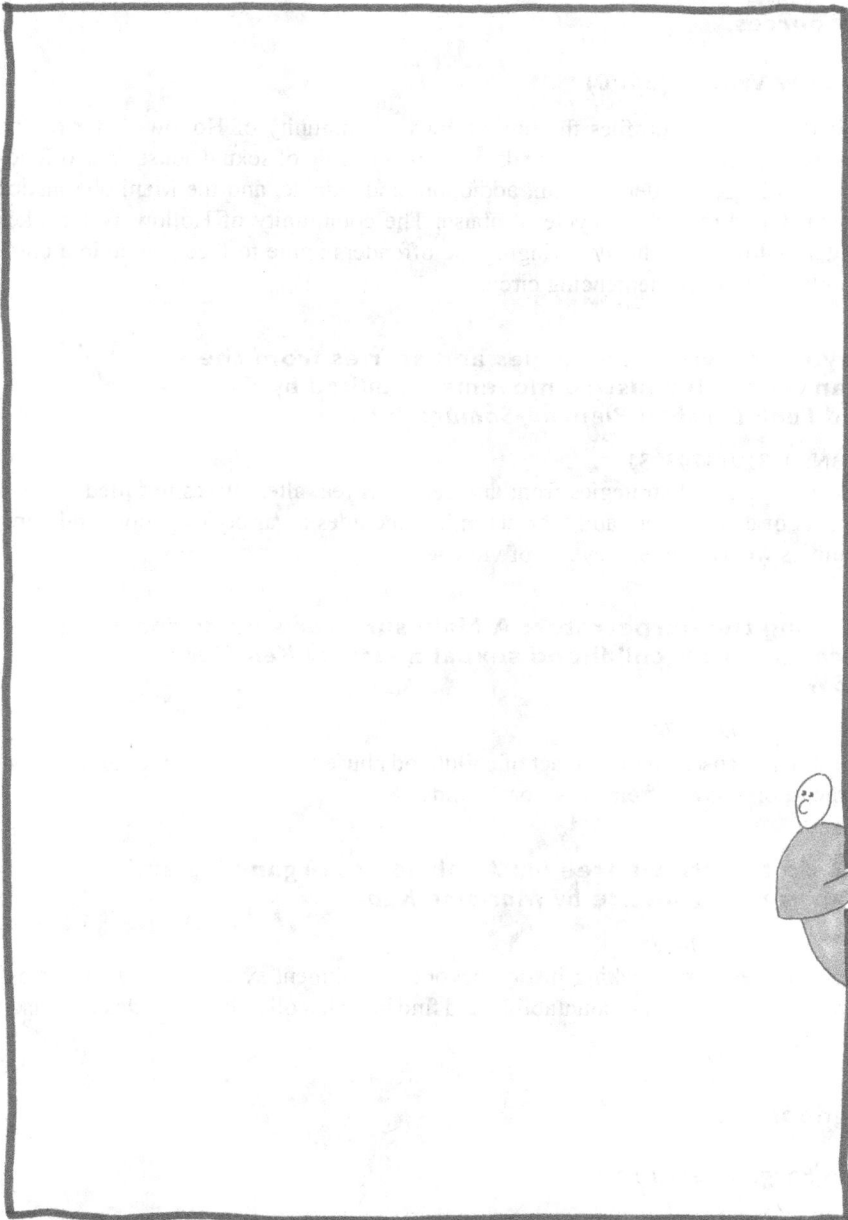

For A4 and printable versions of this worksheet, visit www.jeremysachs.com

Resources

Hollow Water (2000)

This documentary profiles the tiny Ojibway community of Hollow Water on the shores of Lake Winnipeg as it deals with an epidemic of sexual abuse. The offenders left a legacy of denial, pain, addiction, and suicide, and the Manitoba justice system failed to end the cycle of abuse. The community of Hollow Water takes matters into its own hands, bringing the offenders home to face justice in a community healing and sentencing circle.

Beyond survival: Strategies and stories from the transformative justice movement, edited by Ejeris Dixon and Leah Lakshmi Piepzna-Samarasinha

ISBN: 9781913743031
This book puts TJ strategies front and centre as real alternatives to failed modern models of confinement and 'correction'. It includes a variety of people and communities working to end cycles of violence.

Evicting the perpetrator: A Male survivor's guide for recovery from childhood sexual abuse by Ken Singer, MSW

ISBN: 9781929657469
This book focuses on the impact of childhood abuse and how to reduce and remove perpetrators' power from survivors' minds.

We do this 'til we free us: Abolitionist organizing and transforming justice by Mariame Kaba

ISBN-10 1642594288
This book explores seeking justice beyond punishment systems to transform our approach to harm and accountability and find hope in collective struggles for prison abolition.

Signposting

The Forgiveness Project

While not exclusively focused on men, the Forgiveness Project uses real-life stories to explore forgiveness, reconciliation, and conflict resolution. They work with both victims and perpetrators, including those in prison settings.

Eventbrite

www.eventbrite.co.uk
The Eventbrite website hosts a variety of many events and groups based around particular interests or identities. You can search events involving specific hobbies, such as book clubs or running groups, or specific communities, such as immigrant or BIPOC communities. It may be a good first step to finding safe social spaces.

Transform Justice

www.transformjustice.org.uk
This organisation aims to create a fairer, more humane and more effective justice system. They focus on promoting restorative justice, advocating for systemic reforms, and reducing reliance on incarceration.

Black Lives Matter UK (BLMUK)

blacklivesmatter.uk
BLMUK addresses systemic racism and violence against Black communities. They work on various fronts, including advocacy, education, and community support, to combat racial injustice and promote TJ principles.

Restorative Justice for All (RJ4All)

https://rj4all.org
RJ4All works to promote restorative justice principles and practices. They provide community-based programmes, training, and support to help individuals and communities resolve conflict and heal from harm.

Notes

1 Mia Mingus, 'Transformative justice: A brief description', Transform Harm, 11 January 2009. Transform Harm, 1 January 2023. https://transformharm.org/tj_resource/transfo rmative-justice-a-brief-description, accessed 2 August 2024.
2 Name changed.
3 'Male childhood sexual abuse', *The Trauma Talks Podcast*, series 1, episode 2 (Apple Podcasts, 30 June 2020). https://podcasts.apple.com/gb/podcast/1-2-the-trauma-talks-male-childhood-sexual-abuse/id1517405491?i=1000480875439, accessed 5 August 2024.
4 Angela Davis, *Are Prisons Obsolete?* (New York: Seven Stories Press, 2003).
5 Cindy Blackstock and Michael J. Enright, 'The circle process and restorative justice: Practicing traditional Aboriginal conflict resolution in contemporary settings', *Journal of Social Work Practice* 12, no. 1 (1998): 9–22.
6 INCITE! Women of Color Against Violence, 'Home', 2024. https://incite-national.org, accessed 29 May 2024.

7   INCITE! Women of Color Against Violence (ed.), *The Revolution Will Not Be Funded: Beyond the non-Profit Industrial Complex* (Cambridge, MA: South End Press, 2007).

8   Ministry of Justice, *The End-To-End Rape Review Report on Findings and Actions* (HM Government: 18 June 2021; updated 20 August 2021).

9   Betsy Stanko (OBE), *Operation Soteria Bluestone Year 1 Report 2021–2022* (London: UK Home Office, 15 December 2022). www.gov.uk/government/publications/operation-soteria-year-one-report, accessed 2 August 2024.

Chapter 12

For the allies

Chapter Contents

Trauma-informed therapist

I'm Matt. I am a trauma-informed therapist working with survivors across five male prisons. I work with victim-survivors and survivors who perpetrate violence.

For me, being aware that working with these cohorts can lead to us developing compassion fatigue and experiencing moral injury is essential. When working with survivors who are prisoners, you aren't only hearing about the original traumas they experienced at the hands of their abusers. You are hearing about their mistakes and choices that have led them to where they are sat before you. You are hearing their justifications that jar with your own moral compass. You are witnessing survivors who have had to survive experiences that are often painful to hear.

But that isn't all. Because, when working with survivors in prison, you are hearing and often witnessing society's failures. Of an education system that gave up on them. A care system that abused them. A criminal justice system that fails them. And a prison system that often retraumatises them. The survivors are responsible for their choices, but their choices are often limited by the societies and communities that failed them.

It can be difficult to be in that environment and not feel your compassion slipping away from you. It is difficult to witness injustice and not feel morally injured by it. Be sure to maintain your awareness of how you are coping and how you are taking care of yourself.

Matt Metcalf

DOI: 10.4324/9781003423331-12

From the beginning, my goal has been to reflect my therapeutic voice in this book as closely as possible. I wanted to the survivors reading it to hear a friendly, professional tone, akin to what you would experience if we were sitting opposite each other, having a conversation. I also aimed to create a feeling of authentic support for the allies of male survivors who are reading this book. I strove to convey a tone and language in this book that aligned with who I am as a therapist and as an individual navigating my own journey, difficult experiences, and attempts to foster connections with others. However, as the book progressed and my research into male survivors' experiences deepened, my tone began to shift from friendly and professional. Anger started to seep into my writing. Friends and colleagues who read early drafts noticed this change, often pointing out that certain sections didn't sound like my voice or that the tone seemed angry. They were right. When I went back to rewrite those sections, I was often surprised by how emotional my words became without my realising it.

In hindsight, I found two main reasons for this. First, dreams and memories from my past resurfaced as I was writing certain chapters. I'd wake up at night feeling deep shame, or I'd find myself irritable during the day. I often felt the urge to revert to old, unsustainable coping strategies from my past. Even from the safe position I lived in now, the corrosive power of sexual abuse affected me in ways I wasn't fully conscious of, leading anger and resentment to find their way onto the page. Second, I felt increasing anger at how society fails male survivors. I was angry at the families who failed to protect survivors, at the criminal justice system that dismissed and persecuted some survivors and at healthcare professionals who pathologise men's identities or diminish their experiences. The social and health inequalities experienced by male survivors from different backgrounds are undeniable. My anger at these injustices spilled onto the page.

There is, of course, a place for this anger. I never want to censor strong emotions or imply that anger is inherently bad. I also don't want to diminish anger about social injustice – it is important. However, I intended this book to acknowledge the pain and barriers male survivors may face without letting it become all-consuming. Looking back, managing my own challenging emotions and appropriate anger at social injustice has been one of the biggest challenges of the writing process.

Why am I telling you this? Because it's crucial for people who support survivors to recognise the emotional power of this subject matter – not just as you read this book, but as you continue supporting survivors. The insidiousness of sexual abuse can infiltrate survivors' lives without our noticing, and the sheer outrage over the treatment of some survivors can create an all-consuming anger that leaves little room for anything else. Supporting survivors brings you close to some of the most traumatic experiences in their lives. It can also awaken your own traumatic past, even unconsciously. I failed to notice this happening to myself while I wrote parts of this book. I relied on clinical and peer supervision, along with the support of colleagues, to help me recognise and process my emotions.

It is especially important to recognise the potential for emotional overwhelm because, I suspect, some allies reading this book may not only care for a survivor but may also have survived some form of abuse or relational trauma themselves. It's not uncommon for professionals to take an interest in sexual abuse due to some personal connection or experience. It's also not uncommon for male survivors to be in relationships with other survivors. Many allies reading this book may be balancing support for a survivor with looking after themselves. For those of us with trauma in our past, taking on the role of a wounded healer can take significant energy.

12.1   The wounded healer

Carl Jung was a Swiss psychiatrist and psychoanalyst. In 1951, he introduced the term *wounded healer*.[1] It's a great term because you likely already have an idea of what it means, even if it is new to you. While you may care for a survivor or survivors, you are likely also acutely aware of your own wounds or, to use more contemporary language, traumas. Jung believed that our own pain and struggles are the best possible training for healing others, and he eventually argued that only the wounded physician can heal effectively. There is truth in this. Clients often tell me that they'd like to train to become counsellors, psychotherapists, or clinical psychologists but worry they wouldn't be able because of their own mental health challenges, not realising that their curiosity about and willingness to interrogate their mental health uniquely qualifies them for work in this field.

Since Jung, the idea of the wounded healer has been discussed everywhere from holistic healing to academic research circles. In 2006, researcher and therapist Alison Barr's master's thesis, 'An investigation into the extent to which psychological wounds inspire counsellors and psychotherapists to become wounded healers...' found that '73.9% of therapists have experienced one or more wounding experiences leading to career choice'. She goes on:

> [T]he exact causes of the wounds vary enormously. The main categories are abuse, family life as a child, mental ill-health (own), social, family life as an adult, bereavement, mental ill-health (others), life threatening, physical ill-health (others), physical ill-health (own), and, other.[2]

People often care for others because it gives them a sense of wellbeing and purpose. Connecting with others is a fundamental aspect of being human, and supporting others is one of the most profound experiences we can share. Caregivers may attempt to heal themselves by supporting others or find that, in supporting others, they are able to repress their own pain for a while. Some individuals may have grown up around people whom they tried to help or heal but were unable to due to age or circumstance, and therefore seek to heal and support people now.

As allies, it's possible for our own traumas to resurface from the depth of our unconscious, simply because we are close to another person's traumatic experiences. Sometimes we may notice this, and at other times, it may come out in fatigue, anger, apathy, numbness, or frustration. I've spoken to allies, both health-care professionals and those who support loved ones, about some of the impacts of giving their support. See if you can relate to some of them:

- **Emotional impact.** Allies of survivors may feel sadness, anger, or frustration over the survivor's pain and the injustices they face. While this is a natural response, it can be a challenge if it leads us to become overwhelmed. It can also act as a justification to ignore our own feelings, meaning we repress our emotions and solely acknowledge those of the people we care for.
- **Secondary trauma.** Exposure to traumatic stories can lead to secondary or vicarious trauma, causing stress and emotional fatigue. It is common to be deeply affected by stories of sexual abuse because of how deeply shameful, secretive, and damaging the abuse can be. This can be hard to spot as an ally, since the sexual abuse didn't happen to us.
- **Guilt or shame.** Difficultly prioritising self-care over caring for a survivor, particularly if we feel the survivor 'had it worse' or struggles more with their trauma. Allies may feel like we need to be constantly 'on call' to support survivors, and if we prioritise ourselves or try and create boundaries, we may feel guilt or even shame. Many allies acknowledge the importance of self-care generally, but fail to make it a priority for ourselves.
- **Empathy fatigue.** Constant empathy for survivors' experiences can lead us to feel emotional exhaustion or numbness, called *empathy fatigue*. It can be difficult to admit that that our ability to empathise can become diminished or reduced, particularly if we care deeply about the survivor. We may catch ourselves being short-tempered and resentful, leading back to shame or to apathy, where we end our emotional investment in caring for others and simply go through the motions of caring.
- **Becoming enmeshed with the survivor.** Some allies identify with the survivor's struggle so strongly we can become enmeshed with them, forming an 'us against the world' outlook with the survivor. This can develop between survivors and loved ones, friends and therapists. We may feel like we are the only person who really 'gets it', and our existence becomes wrapped up in the survivor's, and vice versa. Boundaries melt away, and survivor and ally become mutually energised by the enmeshed relationship. Such relationships often feel good, making us feel seen and understood, particularly if we have our own wounds and traumas. However, they can be exhausting to maintain. They leave little space for other people and often lack boundaries, potentially resulting in a rift in the relationship.
- **Detachment from our own needs.** Some allies are so good at responding to the survivor's needs that it becomes second nature. We anticipate what the survivor will need and are quick to respond to requests for help and support. Allies often seem unfazed by this, happy to give our time to support someone we care for. However, allies who seem to effortlessly help others have often learned how

to do so from a young age. We learned how to be so caring and responsive to somebody else's needs because a parent, caregiver, or loved one in their past positioned us as a carer, potentially before we were old enough to have a full sense of our own needs. For these allies, caring for others feels like the most normal thing in the world. However, this can become problematic when our own needs come bubbling up, often triggered by a major life event, such as a bereavement, completing higher education or work, having children, or ending a relationship. Life suddenly becomes overwhelming, and the caring role becomes unsustainable.

It can be a delicate challenge to be aware of our own wounds while caring for others, especially when caring for men. Social pressures to avoid appearing weak or burdensome can isolate men and make them hard to reach. Allies must show care without shaming survivors or making them feel their needs are too much. At the same time, we must also prioritise our own emotions and personal trauma. Finding boundaries that work for both ally and survivor is an important part of maintaining a sustainable, compassionate, and caring relationship.

At the heart of effective care lies the art of active listening. While this may sound straightforward, it demands significant effort in practice. Revisiting the basics, for example, by refining listening skills, holds immense value. It's important to acknowledge that mastering these skills isn't just a one-time endeavour; it requires ongoing dedication and self-reflection. Even seasoned professionals can find renewed insight by revisiting foundational techniques and adapting them to the unique context of supporting male survivors. Revisiting these skills through an intersectional lens can provide us with an opportunity to identify our own conscious or unconscious biases. This is important because caring for male survivors can involve all sorts of prejudice; spotting our own can prevent us from further isolating men who need support. Further, actively and authentically listening with our whole being is a good way to check in with ourselves, identifying whether our own wounds are being activated and if we need some self-care.

12.2   Actively listening to survivors

Frequently, when someone we care about experiences pain or faces injustice or abuse, our instinct is to spring into action mode. Much like we would when tending to a child's scraped knee, we rush to soothe, clean the broken skin and apply a plaster to keep the wound free from infection. Addressing a physical wound calls for immediate action. It is an effective and appropriate way to respond to a hurt child. Allies, may attempt the same response for those survivors we care for, springing into action mode to combat the powerlessness and injustice of sexual abuse. We yearn to help our loved one, whose sexual agency was stripped away, reclaim their sense of power. We may devise plans to involve the authorities, seek revenge or research coping strategies. In our efforts to support survivors, we may grapple with our own feelings of helplessness and vulnerability in the face of their overwhelming trauma.

However, when survivors of sexual abuse confide in allies, they don't necessarily want or need the same action-oriented response that soothes a child's physical hurt. In fact, such a response might inadvertently exacerbate a survivor's distress. Allies may feel inadequate when survivors share their abuse stories, finding that our attempts to help only seem to worsen the situation. There can be, of course, a time for action mode, but allies can only gauge whether or not it is appropriate through active listening.

Carl Rogers, who I mentioned in Chapter 10, emphasised the importance of active listening within therapeutic relationships, arguing it was a key component to therapy's facilitation of personal growth and change. He believed that when humans feel listened to, empathised with and accepted, they are able to develop and grow.[3] Rogers outlined several key components of active listening, and I've listed some of them here that are key to supporting survivors. As you read through them, you may wish to consider three things: how you might incorporate them into your allyship, how they might highlight any unconscious bias on your part and what they suggest about your own traumas.

Empathy

Rogers stressed the significance of empathic understanding, in which the listener endeavours to truly grasp the other person's perspective, feelings, and experiences without judgement or bias. When we listen to survivors' stories, whether it's the first time or the hundredth, it's important that we pay attention to how we are feeling. Our ability to empathise is often impaired when we are emotionally distracted. These distractions can come in various forms: perhaps we've heard a similar story before and feel we understand; perhaps we start wondering what we can do or say next to help. We may feel self-conscious and unsure of what to do with our bodies while listening. We might experience boredom or distraction or feel an urge to share our own painful story.

These thoughts and feelings can be loud and obvious or subtle and quiet. They often indicate that the survivor's story is provoking a reaction within us, even on an unconscious level. Such reactions can impair our ability to fully empathise and may be early signs of empathy fatigue or secondary trauma. Being mindful of our own emotional state while listening helps us remain present and supportive, ensuring that we provide the best possible care and understanding to survivors. It's also important to be cautious of feeling like 'we get it', particularly with survivors whose identity is different from ours. While we might have similar experiences to the survivor, our experiences may take on different meanings depending on our culture, identity, relationship to masculinity, or previous trauma. Surviving similar trauma doesn't necessarily mean a survivor feels the same way about it as you.

Unconditional positive regard

Unconditional positive regard involves accepting and valuing another person without conditions or judgement, fostering an atmosphere of trust and openness. This can be challenging to achieve or maintain when survivors share experiences that are difficult for us to fully understand. For instance, I have sat with allies who struggle to comprehend why the survivor they are supporting attended a chemsex party, chatted with someone online, or behaved in ways they didn't expect. When we encounter lifestyles or identities that are unfamiliar to us (even in people we know and love), it can take time for us to process and understand this new information.

Having unconditional positive regard means respecting and valuing another person's agency. Our response to survivors and their stories can reveal a lot about our own biases and perspectives. If you find yourself feeling uncomfortable with a survivor's situation or environment, it might indicate more about your own views than it does about them. For example, feeling uneasy about a survivor's sexual practices may suggest a need to examine your own personal biases or prejudices. This doesn't mean you should compromise your beliefs, but it does mean that you may need to do some work to acknowledge that others' beliefs and choices are equally as valid as your own. As allies, we don't always need to fully understand every aspect of a survivor's identity or choices. However, we do need to respect them and strive to understand as much of them as possible. It is impossible to authentically support a survivor of abuse or rape if we are simultaneously judging them for their actions or identity.

Reflection

Reflective listening involves paraphrasing or summarising the speaker's words to demonstrate understanding and encourage further exploration of their thoughts and feelings. This is one of the first skills therapists learn. As trainees, therapists practise listening and reflecting, using the same language and summarising each other's stories. It's a valuable skill, and for allies, it can be incredibly helpful. Listening for specific language and reflecting it back not only shows we are listening and understanding, but it also reflects back to survivors the hard work they put into communicating something extremely difficult. Particularly for some men, finding the emotional language to describe their feelings can be challenging. The act of saying, 'I was abused' or 'I was raped' requires tremendous bravery and effort, which often goes overlooked. Male survivors have shared with me how those words feel forming in their mouths: surreal, unnatural, heavy, as if saying them will trigger some awful punishment or cause their world to crumble. In reflecting the same language, we communicate that we have heard the survivor and confirm that the world (and us, their allies) hasn't crumbled around them.

I have found that occasionally asking what specific words mean to individual survivors can be beneficial. If a survivor says they feel angry, I might ask, 'What does the word *angry* mean to you?' This helps the survivor unpack complex emotions in a slow, safe way while giving me additional insight into their choice of words. This technique helps me better understand the language male survivors use and, because abuse can feel like the most unspeakable experience a person can endure, it can also add more vocabulary to describe something that has felt indescribable, defusing some of the shame. Reflective listening requires a light touch. It's important not to interrupt or disrupt the bigger picture, but occasionally pausing to probe words' meanings for the survivor can bridge a gap in experience or identity that is worth exploring.

Nonverbal communication

Rogers recognised the importance of nonverbal cues, such as body language and facial expressions, in conveying empathy and understanding. While this may seem obvious at first, nonverbal communication can have different meanings for different individuals. Thinking about nonverbal communication can also encourage us to pay attention to what is going on in our bodies, which can help us understand our past wounds.

Consider eye contact, for example. When working with survivors, I might close my eyes or look down instead of making eye contact. This communicates my focus on the story while helping to alleviate the potential shame some survivors may feel when disclosing sensitive or stigmatised experiences. For some survivors, such as autistic men, eye contact may feel uncomfortable and make them feel pressure to mask – to meet my eyes when they'd rather not. This is a lot of additional pressure to put on autistic survivors, who may feel they need to hide their autism or manage my social expectations of eye contact while also discussing their abuse.

Other survivors may experience dissociative episodes as they retell traumatic events. I've worked with men whose episodes can be so intense that they feel the need to get out of their chair and sit on the floor. In response, I mirror them, putting aside my own chair and sitting on the ground, maintaining the same distance between us. In being mindful of these nonverbal cues and adapting to the needs of each survivor, we can create a more supportive and understanding environment where they can share their experiences. If some mirroring actions, such as sitting on the floor or avoiding eye contact, can feel counterintuitive, pay attention to your inner sense of connection. Often, this is a good indication of whether you are doing effective nonverbal communication or not.

When we think about what our bodies communicate to others, it's worth also thinking about what our bodies communicate to ourselves. Pay attention to any physical sensations you experience while talking with survivors. You might feel fidgety, have an impulse to pick up your phone, or experience aches and pains. It's easy to chastise ourselves for being distracted by these things, but asking ourselves, *What about supporting the survivor in this moment made me distracted?* can produce useful information about our unconscious emotions or the survivor's discomfort.

Survivor-led active listening

In addition to Rogers' active listening skills, I want to add that active listening is *survivor-led*. While the term *active listening skills* implies the conversation is led by the person speaking, it's worth thinking about ways to facilitate letting male survivors lead. Following are eight ways to consider making your support survivor-led:

1. **Believe survivors.** Often, when male survivors disclose, their experiences are dismissed. It is crucial for allies to offer them something the rest of the world often hasn't: belief. By simply believing men and letting them be experts in their own experience, you provide a powerful form of support.

   On your first hearing of an abuse story, there may be aspects of the that story don't immediately make sense to you, or you may feel the need to question some details. These questions can wait. Asking investigative questions too soon can negatively impact survivors as they share their stories, because they may feel that you don't believe them. If you need more details for any reason, you can address them later. Believing male survivors is not only important, but it can be considered radical in a world where they are rarely believed. Your belief can make a profound difference in their healing journey.

2. **Ask open questions.** Asking questions that cannot be answered with a simple 'yes' or 'no' encourages more detailed and elaborate responses. These questions typically start with words like 'how', 'why', 'what', 'describe to me', or 'tell me about'. They are important because they gently support the survivor in describing their story or feelings in detail.

3. **Check in with how survivors are feeling and whether they feel safe.** It can be helpful to ask survivors about their emotional state, ensuring they feel safe in the moment. It can be easy for some survivors to overshare or work themselves into an unsafe emotional state that they may not want to be in. Asking survivors to check in with their feelings is a simple way of supporting them.

   Be careful however, that you don't use technique to censor survivors' feelings if you become uncomfortable with their strong emotions. We can be tempted to say something like, 'This conversation doesn't feel safe for you', when we feel out of our depth. Allow survivors strong emotions, even if they are uncomfortable, and let them decide whether or not a conversation is safe.

4. **Reassuring them that they are in control.** Sexual abuse survivors have endured an experience where their control was removed. Affirming to survivors that they have power and authority over conversations about their abuse can help them feel empowered and secure. Achieving this can be as simple as saying, 'You tell me what you want to talk about', or 'I'm just here to listen to whatever you want to say'.

5. **Asking what they need from you.** Asking what specific support or assurance survivors need from you ensures survivors' needs are understood and addressed. Often, survivors respond that they don't know, and this is okay; the question itself communicates your care and the survivor's control.

6. **Recognising Intersectionality.** As we've seen throughout this book, understanding the ways in which survivors' experiences can be shaped by multiple intersecting identities and society's views on these identities can influence our approach to their trauma and their ability to heal. Recognising intersectionality impacts our ability to understand male survivors' experiences. Even if a survivor has a different background to you, you can still offer support that gains value as you become more aware of the intersecting elements of the survivor's identity and your own biases. Regardless of your own identity, you may want to reflect on the following areas:

   a) **Demonstrating cultural and social sensitivity.** It is important that allies educate ourselves on the cultural, social, and historical contexts that can affect survivors differently. Seek out books, events, or courses to try to avoid putting the burden of your education on the survivor. Working on your cultural and social sensitivity and education away from your supporting role can free you up to focus on the caring relationship when you are with survivors.

   b) **Acknowledging power dynamics.** Be mindful of how systemic power imbalances impact survivors and how your own position with survivors might mirror systemic imbalances. This may look different depending on your relationship with the survivor, be it friend, relative, or therapist. Different dynamics will affect your relationship with survivors and their trust and comfort levels.

   c) **Respecting autonomy.** It is important to respect survivors' choices and give them control over their own healing. This may mean their recovery looks different from how you want it to look. Sexual abuse removes survivors' autonomy, and when allies dictate how survivors ought to heal, it can feel like we are disregarding their autonomy again. In addition, recovering from sexual abuse is rarely linear, and survivors may need to make choices that seem counterintuitive or differ from choices you would make. As long as they are not seriously harming themselves or others, the general rule is to trust survivors as experts in their own recovery; they are likely doing the best they can at that moment in time.

7. **Being aware of your own internalised toxic masculinity.** This can be difficult for allies supporting men. Chances are, from the second you were born, regardless of your gender, you've been told how 'real men' should behave, think, dress, and feel. Allies not only need to be aware of how toxic masculinity can impact survivors of any gender, but we should also work towards recognising the ways our own biases might impact our ability to be good allies.

8. **Knowing yourself.** Male survivors often want to have conversations about identity, gender, sex, abuse, complex power relations, and difficult family dynamics. Male survivors come from all backgrounds, lifestyles, and identities. Allies who don't examine our own relationships with these topics, identities, and ways of being risk judging or misunderstanding survivors, raising a significant barrier to authentic support and connection.

If a survivor tells you something about their abuse story, culture, or lifestyle that makes you feel uncomfortable or judgemental, take note and reflect on why the topic makes you feel that way. Ask yourself why you feel uncomfortable and what in your life has influenced or informed this discomfort. Do you hold beliefs that may be problematic or impact your ability to authentically empathise and show unconditional positive regard? This sounds like a simple question, but answering it requires us to examine our beliefs and upbringing and, possibly, some scary parts of ourselves we'd rather ignore. This practice should also be habitual rather than a one-off. This will allow us to detach ourselves from scary beliefs or emotions and foster a deeper sense of connection and understanding with the survivor as a person, rather than letting our preconceived ideas or unconscious biases dictate the relationship.

I asked Anna Linde, a certified sex coach with an MS in sexology, how she balances paying attention to her own body and trauma with her work with male survivors. A transracial adoptee born in Brazil and raised in Sweden by white parents, Linde uses an intersectional approach in every session of her work. As she told me,

> We ask for these men to summon the courage to be vulnerable and trust us. They need our authenticity, and we need to understand exactly what we are asking them to do. We need to lead by example, embody courage, empathy and hold the space for the externalisation of their pain. My capacity to embody this level of courage demands me to stay connected, with myself and the survivor. The impulse to give in to the triggers awakened within while listening to the survivor describe the trauma is easy to succumb to. I feel these triggers as stiffness in my shoulders, tightness in my chest and a clenched jaw. If I fail to stay grounded in these moments, I also fail to provide a sense of safety in our intimate and vulnerable conversation as well as I fail to share their pain. It is crucial that I ground myself throughout our conversation and keep the presence and authenticity of our meeting.[4]

Taking action

As we've discussed, allies can be tempted to spring into action with male survivors, but doing so often means missing the opportunity to sit with them and make them feel truly heard. When it *is* time for action, we need to be led by survivors. It's important to avoid letting our internal rescuer (see Chapter 2, page 54) take charge and act in the ways we believe are best. We may feel a desire to march to the police station and demand justice. However, the appropriate action can be as simple as asking survivors when and where they'd like to meet again to talk more.

Taking action is not the same as taking control. Giving survivor-led, practical support is essential. For example, an ally may think reporting abuse to the police is the best course of action while the survivor does not. Because sexual abuse removes victims' agency, it is important that we do not inadvertently remove their agency again by trying to help. If you are in doubt or start to feel overwhelmed, return to the basics of active listening. I do this regularly! When abuse narratives get complicated, my own feelings start getting too loud, or I notice a seed of discomfort in reaction to someone else's story, I internally return to the practice of active listening.

12.3 Creating a care plan

Creating a care plan can get you started in thinking about how to support yourself while you support survivors. Even if you never return to your plan, the process of creating one can encourage you to take stock, identifying resources, spotting vulnerabilities and creating strategies that can provide you with tools to meet future challenges. The best care plans are tailored to the individual's needs and circumstances; what works for one person may not work for another, and a coping strategy that works for you one week may not work the next. It's best to approach care plans with flexibility, changing and adding to them as you learn more about yourself.

Reflective activity

This activity consists of things you may wish to consider when devising your care plan. It's written with survivors and allies in mind. Don't be afraid to make it your own, disregarding areas that don't apply to you and adding things I didn't. This plan is meant to help you think about how to manage your self-care, either to cope with your own trauma or support survivors in your life. Use a blank sheet in this book, or grab a pen and paper, and consider how these seven categories might help with your self-care.

1. Self-assessment

Consider your challenges and symptoms. This may include diagnoses and clinical language, such as depression, anxiety, complex post-traumatic stress disorder (cPTSD), personality disorders, etc, or it might involve more abstract language (see Chapter 3, page 48). Identify situations or circumstances that activate, trigger, or stress these symptoms, including birthdays, travel, busy environments, being alone, conflict, or specific smells, modes of travel, people, or geographical areas.

This list might grow as you learn more about yourself and what activates your symptoms; it might also shrink as you become desensitised to certain triggers. This doesn't mean that they stop being upsetting, but that your response to them becomes less severe.

2.   Current coping strategies

List your current coping strategies for your mental health. Try to list everything without judgement about whether it is sustainable or unsustainable (see Chapter 10 on coping, page 191). This may be difficult, requiring you to examine your relationship to things you have complicated feelings about, such as pornography, nicotine, food, drugs, or self-harm.

Try to find a balance among your coping strategies. Consider which strategies are healthier for you than others. This is often harder than it first seems. For example, a glass of wine or a chocolate bar may be just what you want to cope in a stressful moment, but in excess, these strategies become unsustainable. The goal is to add sustainable strategies to this list through self-reflection and support, rather than focusing on reducing unsustainable strategies. If you feel that your list only has unsustainable strategies, you might set a goal to discover new ways of coping.

3.   Clear goals

Setting clear goals, whether long- or short-term, can be helpful. Short-term goals are achievable within a few weeks or months. They may include things like not letting a family member cause you a panic attack this holiday season or checking out counselling directories to make a short list of potential therapists. Long-term goals are broader and may take longer to achieve. They may include finding and committing to attending support groups or managing anxiety more effectively.

4.   Formal support

Formal support means something different to each individual depending on their identity and circumstances. For some people, it means seeking medication from a doctor and finding a mental health professional to work with. For others, it means peer-led support, such as a survivor group. Importantly, this support is separate from friends or family who you may confide in. Once you have found formal support, schedule and maintain a regular practice with it, staying accountable to yourself and to your formal support system.

5. Social support system

Let trusted people in your life know when your mental health is causing challenges. It is important to communicate with the people who care for you, even if it is hard. If it's difficult for you, start small. Experiment with disclosing little things and reflecting on how it goes. If it goes well, disclose a little more or ask explicitly for the support you need. Taking small steps can help us learn what to expect from people and to protect our feelings if people disappoint us.

7. Wellbeing

- Moving your body. Not everyone wants or is able to create an exercise routine, but regular physical activity, whatever that means to you, is an important way to enhance your overall wellbeing. Try different activities, from stretching or 'chair yoga' to walking around the block or engaging in sport. Moving your body can soothe anxiety and depression, as well as boosting physical health.
- Diet. Maintaining a balanced diet can be challenging. Emotional eating presents unique difficulties. Unlike drugs, we not only need and are expected to consume food, but we find it everywhere from train station shops to social spaces. Much of life revolves around food. Consuming a balance of foods that we like, that make us feel better, and that are good for our body is an ongoing struggle for many people.
- Hydration. Though drinking water is probably the simplest-sounding coping mechanism, so few of us remember to do it. Hydrating throughout the day is important for your health, and you should challenge yourself to stay hydrated. The NHS website advises that we 'should aim to drink 6 to 8 cups or glasses of fluid a day', enough that our urine 'is a clear pale yellow colour'.[5]
- Sleep. Sleep can be difficult for anyone. Though we're often advised to aim for between seven and nine hours of sleep per night, different people need different amounts of sleep. (For instance, my sleep

has fluctuated between four and six hours per night for my entire adult life).

If sleep is challenging for you, try asking yourself what you can control about your sleep habits rather than focusing on the sleep itself. Can you have a restful 30 or 60 minutes before bed? Can you allow yourself more time to wake up well? Can you put practices in place to get rest outside of bedtime, regardless of whether you get any sleep?

8. Coping strategies

Integrating coping strategies into your lifestyle means you have something on hand if an unexpected stressor pops up. There are many coping strategies in this book. Why not experiment with and practise them to find which work for you so you're able to employ them when you're out and about. You might also try researching the following methods:

- Mindfulness and meditation
- Deep breathing exercises
- Relaxation techniques
- Journaling
- Nature exposure

It may also be necessary to devise a plan for times when your coping strategies don't work or you're in a crisis:

- **Recognise crisis signs.** Know the warning signs that you are having a mental health crisis. These are different for everyone. Some people develop physical symptoms such as headaches or eczema, while others may feel manic or become withdrawn. When you are not in crisis, write out a list of warning signs you might look for. It may also help to ask trusted people around you if they have noticed any signs you are in distress that you might add to the list.
- **Emergency contacts.** Keep a list of emergency contacts, including mental health professionals, support organisations, and services. Check which services operate during the workday, public holidays, or 24 hours a day. SurvivorsUK, for example, has a helpline that operates broadly during the day, but the Samaritans mental health helpline is available for 24 hours, 7 days a week. Knowing contacts'

availability ahead of a crisis can be useful, as can identifying trusted friends to call. It may be a good idea to share that you'd like to add them to your crisis plan so they can prepare to offer support, should you need it.

- **Know where supportive items are at all times.** Supportive items are anything we use to keep from disassociating, including a hand cream we like to smell, favourite jumper, song we love, or flavoured sweet. When I ran a youth service, I often gave out Fisherman's Friends, a sweet flavoured with menthol, eucalyptus, and liquorice, first created in 1865. Young people who sometimes dissociated or wanted to self-harm found them a useful grounding tool due to the strong taste.

Review your care plan

Once you've created your care plan, don't assume it won't need to be changed or edited. As we learn new things about ourselves and grow and develop, so do our needs. Checking in with yourself or asking a therapist or friend to help you can be a really important way of looking after yourself, whether you are a survivor of abuse or an ally.

I've heard people say at conferences and talks about male survivors that it takes specially trained experts to effectively work with men who have experienced rape or abuse. I always have a mixed reaction to this. While I absolutely want all survivors to find the support they need and for that support to be from highly skilled professionals, I also know the world doesn't always work that way. Many people who support survivors, either in their personal lives or in therapy rooms, do not have specific training or experiences that label them as 'experts' in men's sexual trauma.

Allies in a relationship with a survivor are often already in the relationship before they learn about the abuse. Some men wait decades to disclose to their allies or attend therapy for months or years before they feel safe enough to share an abuse story. What are allies who have already developed a meaningful relationship with male survivors meant to do? End the relationship? Attend years of intensive training? Tell survivors that we could support them before we knew about the abuse, but now we know about it, we're not skilled enough to do so? These options seem impractical at best and damaging at worst.

One of this book's main themes is connection, because in my experience, authentic connection is the antidote to the pain, shame, and isolation of sexual abuse. In these pages, I encourage male survivors to take risks, be proactive, and make new connections. This is where allies can help. Reaching out authentically to survivors and listening to and believing them may be the best support we can offer.

While it absolutely helps to have relevant education, expertise, and experience, it is just as important to have an authentic relationship with the survivor and ourselves. We achieve this by getting to know ourselves, our conscious or unconscious biases, our relationship to past trauma and taking our rest and boundaries seriously. Like a lot of the advice in this book, this is a constant practice rather than a one-off act. Some of the most authentic and impactful healers I know are honest with themselves first in order to be authentic with others. By following their example, allies can offer valuable support to the survivors in our lives.

A Postcard To Your Future

As you reach the end of this book, it's helpful to start thinking about your future self.

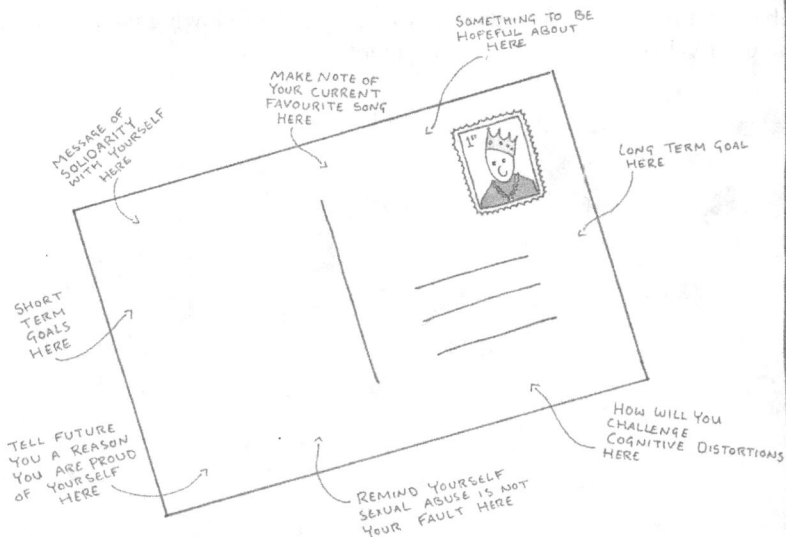

In this exercise, write a message to your future self. Grab a postcard or draft an email, and note down everything you'll be taking away from this book and this moment in your life. Include serious insights, like new ways of thinking or important facts you've learned, as well as more personal reflections, like your favourite songs right now. If you write on a postcard, put it away and set a reminder to read it in 6 or 12 months. If it's an email, schedule it to send to yourself in 6 or 12 months. Remind your future self what's important to remember now!

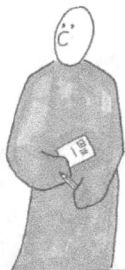

www.jeremysachs.com   @JeremySachs_

For A4 and printable versions of this worksheet, visit www.jeremysachs.com

www.jeremysachs.com   @JeremySachs_

For A4 and printable versions of this worksheet, visit www.jeremysachs.com

Notes

1 Carl Jung, *Fundamental Questions of Psychotherapy* (Princeton, NJ: Princeton University Press, 1951).
2 Alison Barr, 'An investigation into the extent to which psychological wounds inspire counsellors and psychotherapists to become wounded healers, the significance of these wounds on their career choice, the causes of these wounds and the overall significance of demographic factors', iii. Available via The Green Rooms, https://thegreenrooms.net/wounded-healer-research-for-counsellors-and-psychotherapists, accessed 2 August 2024.
3 Carl R. Rogers and Rosalind F. Dymond (eds.), *Client-Centered Therapy: Its Current Practice, Implications, and Theory* (Boston: Houghton Mifflin, 1951).
4 Personal interview correspondence, July 2024.
5 'Water, drinks and hydration', National Health Service (NHS), last reviewed 15 December 2021. www.nhs.uk/live-well/eat-well/food-guidelines-and-food-labels/water-drinks-nutrition, accessed 2 August 2024

A final message to the reader

As I write the final lines of this book, I am thinking about you, reader. I wonder where you are in the world, whether you are a survivor, an ally, or perhaps both. I am curious about your hobbies, interests, relationships, and what brings you joy. I want to know how you define your masculinity: do you embrace traditional values of strength, responsibility, and loyalty, or is your masculinity more fluid, feminine, or non-defined? I like imagining these things because I believe we are all so much more than the trauma we survive.

I hope this book has shown you that healing is not a solitary journey. It requires us to reach out and step out of our comfort zone. If we want our future to be different from our past, we need to expose ourselves to new things. This is often counter-intuitive to the lessons we learn surviving sexual abuse, which teach us to keep our head down and to suspect danger everywhere. It also contradicts what society has taught us about masculinity: that asking for help is weak. Hopefully, society's understandings of masculinity and trauma are evolving; what is true today may not be tomorrow. The same can be said for us: what holds us back today might have less power tomorrow, and what once seemed impossible might now be within our reach. My hope is also that this book contributes to the growing intersectional literature on sexual abuse and that men from all backgrounds and identities find their experiences represented in these pages. My deepest wish is that this book offers validation and strength to those who feel invisible and unheard.

I want to acknowledge the bravery of all survivors who have shared their experiences and identities with me. Your wisdom has guided my writing. I also want to acknowledge your bravery in reading these pages, reader. Facing the painful experiences of sexual abuse is a profound act of courage, particularly for male survivors. It is a genuine privilege to have written this book for you. Thank you.

Appendix 1

All the resources and signposting in one place

Chapter 2

Resources

- *Close to Home* (ISBN: 9780241582978) – by Michael Magee
- The Trauma Talks podcast – by Jeremy Sachs and Katherine Cox

Signposting

- 1in6 – https://1in6.org

Chapter 3

Resources

- *Trauma Is Really Strange* (ISBN: 9781848192935) – by Steve Haines
- *Prejudice, Social Stress, and Mental Health in Lesbian, Gay, and Bisexual Populations: Conceptual Issues and Research Evidence* – by Ilan H. Meyer
- The World Health Organisation created, 'A practical handbook on Adverse Childhood Experiences (ACEs) Delivering prevention, building resilience, and developing trauma-informed systems A resource for professionals and organisations'

Signposting

- PTSD UK – www.ptsduk.org
- Mind – www.mind.org.uk

Chapter 4

Resources

- *Mask Off: Masculinity Redefined* (ISBN: 9780745338743) – by J.J. Bola
- *Sons and Others: On Loving Male Survivors* (ISBN: 9781912489640) – by Tanaka Mhishi

Signposting

- Future Men – https://futuremen.org
- Andy's Man Club – https://andysmanclub.co.uk

Chapter 5

Resources

- *Anxiety Is Really Strange* (ISBN: 9781848193895) – by Steve Haines
- Baby Reindeer (2024) – TV show

Signposting

- CALM – www.thecalmzone.net

Chapter 6

Resources

- *Games People Play* (ISBN 0140027688) – by Eric Berne
- *Families We Choose Lesbians, Gays, Kinship – Between Men – Between Women* (ISBN: 9780231110938) – by Kath Weston
- Pose – a TV show

Signposting

- Tavistock Relationships – https://tavistockrelationships.org
- Relate – www.relate.org.uk
- Relationships Scotland – https://www.relationships-scotland.org.uk
- Mental Health Foundation – www.mentalhealth.org.uk

Chapter 7

Resources

- The Trauma Talks podcast – by Jeremy Sachs and Katherine Cox: Chemsex
- *BDSM and Kink: The Basics* (ISBN 9781032320632) – by Stefani Goerlich and Elyssa Helfer
- I May Destroy You – a TV series by Michaela Coel

Signposting

- Fumble – https://fumble.org.uk
- Terrence Higgins Trust – www.tht.org.uk
- Sex Positivity UK – www.sexpositivityuk.com

Chapter 8

Resources

- *Beyond Betrayal: Taking Charge of Your Life After Boyhood Sexual Abuse* (ISBN-13: 978-0471619109) – by Richard Gartner
- *John Bowlby and Attachment Theory: Makers of Modern Psychotherapy* (ISBN 0415629039) – by Jeremy Holmes
- *Good Will Hunting* (1997) – a film

Signposting

- The ManKind Initiative – https://mankind.org.uk

Chapter 9

Resources

- *The Boy with the Perpetual Nervousness: A Memoir of an Adolescence* (ISBN: 9781509830671) – by Graham Caveney

Signposting

- Crime Stoppers – https://crimestoppers-uk.org
- Rape Crisis England & Wales and Rape Crisis Scotland – https://rapecrisis.org.uk, www.rapecrisisscotland.org.uk

Chapter 10

Resources

- *Shame* – a film
- The Addicted Mind – a Podcast

Signposting

- Action for Addiction – www.actiononaddiction.org.uk
- SMART Recovery – smartrecovery.org.uk
- Release – www.release.org.uk
- Addaction – www.wearewithyou.org.uk

Chapter 11

Resources

- *Hollow Water* documentary: https://www.nfb.ca/film/hollow_water/#
- *Beyond Survival: Strategies and Stories from the Transformative Justice Movement* (ISBN: 9781913743031) – Ejeris Dixon (Editor); Leah Lakshmi Piepzna-Samarasinha (Editor)
- *Evicting the Perpetrator: A Male Survivor's Guide for Recovery from Childhood Sexual Abuse* (ISBN: 9781929657469) – by Ken Singer MSW
- *We Do This 'Til We Free Us: Abolitionist Organizing and Transforming Justice* (ISBN-10 1642594288) – by Mariame Kaba

Signposting

- The Forgiveness Project – www.theforgivenessproject.com
- Eventbrite – www.eventbrite.co.uk
- Transform Justice – www.transformjustice.org.uk
- Black Lives Matter UK (BLMUK) – https://blacklivesmatter.uk
- Restorative Justice for All (RJ4All) – https://rj4all.org

Appendix 2

All exercises and reflective activities

Chapter 8

Building trust – reflective activity: page 167
Managing autistic fatigue and burn out – exercise: page 169

Chapter 9

Why Disclose? – reflective activity/exercise: page 185

Chapter 10

Cognitive distortions – reflective activity: page 196
Urge surfing – exercise: page 205

Chapter 11

Timelines – exercise: page 224

Chapter 12

Creating a care plan – reflective activity: page 240
Postcard to yourself – exercise: page 246

Appendix 3

Emotions wheel

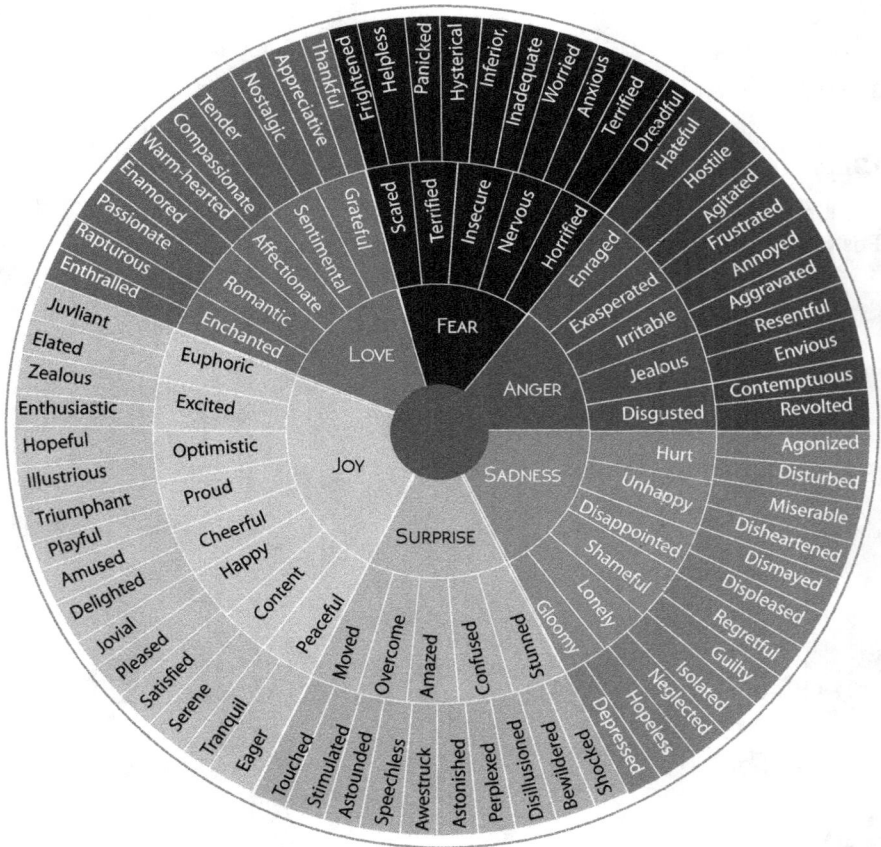

Aimen Yonus/Shutterstock.com

Index

For Product Safety Concerns and Information please contact our EU
representative GPSR@taylorandfrancis.com
Taylor & Francis Verlag GmbH, Kaufingerstraße 24, 80331 München, Germany

9 781032 721903